Financial Management of the Hospital Food Service Department

Faisal A. Kaud

American Hospital Association
840 North Lake Shore Drive
Chicago, Illinois 60611

Library of Congress Cataloging in Publication Data

Kaud, Faisal A.
　　Financial management of the hospital food service department.

　　Bibliography: p.
　　1. Hospitals—Food service—Finance. 2. Hospitals—Business management. I. Title. [DNLM: 1. Financial management. 2. Food service, Hospital—Economics. 3. Food service, Hospital—Organization and administration. WX 168 K21f]
RA975.5.D5K384　1983　　　362.1'76'0681　　83-12238
ISBN 0-87258-411-9

AHA catalog no. 046205

©1983 by the
American Hospital Association
840 North Lake Shore Drive
Chicago, Illinois 60611

All rights reserved. The reproduction or use of this work in any form or in any information storage or retrieval system is forbidden without the express, written permission of the publisher.

Printed in the U.S.A.
2M-9/83-3-0253

American Hospital Association staff:
Audrey Young, Editor, Book Department
Marjorie Weissman, Manager, Book Department
Dorothy Saxner, Director, Division of Books and Newsletters

To Bonnie B. Miller, former senior staff specialist and society director, Department of Patient and Community Services, American Hospital Association, for her leadership, foresight, guidance, and dedication to the American Society for Hospital Food Service Administrators in particular and to hospital food service administration in general.

Contents

List of Figures vii

List of Tables viii

Preface ix

Chapter 1   Financial Data for Management Decision Making and Control 1

Chapter 2   Budgetary Control Process 13

Chapter 3   Capital Investment Analysis 35

Chapter 4   Evaluation of Cost Allocation Methods 47

Chapter 5   Management of the Clinical Dietetics Staff 59

List of Figures

1. Sample Form for Labor Time Report 12
2A-P. Decision Package..21
3. Organizational Chart of Functional Responsibilities in a Food Service Department 29
4. Food Service Department Activity....................................30
5. Example of Priority Ranking..31
6. Sample Form for Financial Reports 32
7. Sample Form for Position Control...................................33
8. Sample Form for Measuring Performance 34
9. Sample Form for Evaluation of Capital Equipment Requests..............45
10. Example of Objectives and Tasks for a Clinical Inpatient Dietitian 67
11. Example of Objectives and Tasks for a Dietetic Technician 68
12. Example of Relative Value Unit Calculations for the Clinical Inpatient Dietitian..69
13. Sample Form for Clinical Dietetics Weekly Status Report 70
14. Sample Form for Diet Status Report 72
15. Sample Report of a Clinical Dietetic Staff's Weekly Activities, Based on Time-Task Allocation Analysis......................................73
16. Sample Report of a Dietitian's Weekly Activities in an Outpatient Nutrition Clinic, Based on Time-Task Allocation Analysis 74
17. Example of a Weekly Activities Budget Study for an Inpatient Clinical Dietetics Department 75

List of Tables

1. Operating Statement for Patient and Nonpatient Activities 2
2. Operating Statement and Revised Budget 4
3. Food Cost Index Work Sheet 7
4. Supply Cost Index Work Sheet 8
5. Present Value of Ordinary Annuity of $1.00, Selected Values 38
6. Earnings at 9.63 Percent on Invested Capital and Recovery of Investment in 10 Years 39
7. Present Net Value with Cash Inflow Discounted at 8 Percent 39
8. Present Net Value with Cash Inflow Discounted at 16 Percent 40
9. Life-Cycle Cost for Meal Assembly Line Replacement: Alternative A 41
10. Present Value of $1.00 Due in N Periods, Selected Values 42
11. Life-Cycle Cost for Meal Assembly Line Replacement: Alternative B 43
12. Summary of Life-Cycle Costs for Alternatives A and B 44
13. Cost Allocation Based on Centralized Food Service Activities as Determined by Meals 50
14. Cost Allocation Based on Centralized Food Service Activities as Determined by Portions 52
15. Labor Costs of Centralized Food Production 53
16. Labor Costs of Cafeteria 55
17. Total Labor Costs of Cafeteria 55
18. Labor Costs of Patient Meal Service 56
19. Total Labor Costs of Patient Meal Service 57
20. Cost Allocation for Cafeteria Based on Meal Equivalent and Operating Expense 57
21. Cost Allocation of Cafeteria Resources 58

Preface

Financial Management of the Hospital Food Service Department has been prepared to assist food service administrators in choosing appropriate methods to evaluate the financial management of their department. Rising health care costs have become the focus of increasing concern among health care administrators and have necessitated a serious, thorough analysis of the financial management of each department.

The primary purpose of this book is to provide food service administrators with the necessary analytical techniques to:

- Review the financial data needed for better decision making
- Outline a budgetary control process whereby predetermined objectives can be evaluated and the specific examination of the food service department can be accomplished
- Demonstrate the applicability of the appropriate capital investment analyses in evaluating the various capital expenditure alternatives
- Review and evaluate cost allocation methods
- Delineate an approach to the management of the clinical dietary staff

The author gratefully acknowledges the contribution of Donna S. Becker, M.S., R.D., assistant director, Clinical Dietetics, University of Wisconsin Hospital and Clinics, Madison, who contributed valuable comments and prepared chapter 5, Management of the Clinical Dietetics Staff. The author wishes to thank members of the clinical dietetics staff at the University of Wisconsin Hospital and Clinics for their assistance and contributions over the years in preparing, implementing, and monitoring the Clinical Dietetics Management Information System, on which chapter 5 was partially based, and members of the secretarial staff for their patient preparation of this document for publication.

The support of the American Society for Hospital Food Service Administrators of the American Hospital Association in the development and preparation of this publication is gratefully acknowledged. Particular appreciation is expressed to Bonnie B. Miller, former senior staff specialist, and Mary D. DeMarco, senior staff specialist, Office of Human Resources-Personal Membership Services, and to Audrey Young for editing the manuscript.

Faisal A. Kaud
Assistant Administrator
University of Wisconsin Hospital
and Clinics

Financial Data for Management Decision Making and Control

Chapter 1

The annual budget of a food service department serves as a plan for the allocation of resources for labor, food, supplies, and other expenses.[1] This allocation of resources enables the food service administrator to organize the department to produce the desired services. The food service administrator then prepares plans to meet the stated objectives of the department as well as the forecast level of activities, such as the number of meals to be served, the number of nutritional assessments to be done, the number of patient visitations, and so forth. In anticipation of these forecast food service activities, the food service administrator schedules employees for work, purchases food and supplies, and orders the preparation of certain foods to meet the published menu. During this process, the department incurs other operating expenses, such as depreciation, office supplies, menus, laundry, repairs, telephone, and so forth.

These operating expenses are recorded on a monthly operating statement that summarizes the cost of providing these services to patients and other customers, compares monthly expenditures with the forecast budget, and highlights areas of compliance and variance. It is customary to conduct an examination of the operating statement on a monthly basis, or as warranted, to ensure compliance with budget guidelines and preestablished objectives and to maintain financial integrity.

The food service administrator examines the overall performance of the department and determines what activities need to be reviewed in order to ameliorate problem areas. In this way, the quality of the decision making can be ascertained. This chapter provides a case study of a food service department's performance, and gives details of the various aspects of this evaluative approach.

Comparison of Financial Operating Data with Budget

In this section the hypothetical hospital food service department's financial operating data are compared with what has been budgeted. Table 1, Operating Statement for Patient and Nonpatient Activities, next page, outlines these five major areas:

1. Patient Days (lines 1-3)

The patient days section provides an overall view of the business volume and outlines increases or decreases in costs. This information shows that the number of actual patient days was 2.6 percent below the budgeted amount, reflecting a decrease of 2,150 patient days. The reduced number of patient days indicates that a lower expenditure is expected in order to maintain costs within the budgetary guidelines.

Clinic visits showed an increase of 5,000 visits, or 3.3 percent, which may have some implication for the level of activity and costs associated with the nutrition clinic. However, further study is required to ascertain the actual level of activity in the nutrition clinic as compared with the budgeted activity in the clinic.

2. Meal Count (lines 4-10)

The meal count section details the actual number of meals served for patients, in the cafeteria, as stipends, and for special functions. It should be noted that the number of

Table 1. Operating Statement for Patient and Nonpatient Activities

Activity	Annual Total Actual	Budget	Variance
1. Patient Days			
2. Patient Days	80,350	82,500	−2.6%
3. Clinic visits	155,000	150,000	+3.3%
4. Meal Count			
5. Patient meals	224,980	231,000	−2.6%
6. Cafeteria meals	124,300	122,925	+1.1%
7. Stipend meals	19,650	19,950	−1.5%
8. Special function	26,225	27,000	−2.9%
9. Other meals	0	0	
10. Total meals	395,155	400,875	−1.4%
11. Operating Expenses			
12. Salary and benefit expenses	$355,000	$344,340	+3.1%
13. Food expenses	$362,750	$349,031	+3.9%
14. Supply expenses	$ 66,250	$ 64,751	+2.3%
15. Other expenses	$ 20,500	$ 21,266	−3.6%
16. Total operating expenses	$804,500	$779,388	+3.2%
17. Less cash receipts	($300,375)	($297,281)	+1.0%
18. Net dietary expenses	$504,125	$482,107	+4.6%
19. Statistical Indicator/Unit Cost per Meal			
20. Salary and benefit expenses	$ 0.90	$ 0.86	+4.6%
21. Food expenses	$ 0.92	$ 0.87	+5.7%
22. Supply expenses	$ 0.17	$ 0.16	+6.2%
23. Other expenses	$ 0.05	$ 0.05	—
24. Total operating expenses	$ 2.04	$ 1.94	+5.1%
25. Less cash receipts	($ 0.76)	($ 0.74)	+2.7%
26. Net cost per meal	$ 1.28	$ 1.20	+6.7%
27. Net cost per patient day	$ 6.27	$ 5.84	+7.4%
28. Productivity Indicators			
29. Meals per hour—paid	5.39	5.63	−4.3%
30. Meals per hour—worked	4.74	4.95	−4.2%
31. Meals per patient day	4.92	4.86	+1.2%

patient meals, stipend meals, and special-function meals declined by 2.6 percent, 1.5 percent, and 2.9 percent, respectively, whereas cafeteria meals increased by 1.1 percent. However, the total number of meals for patient and nonpatient activities declined by 5,720 meals, or 1.4 percent.

3. Operating Expenses (lines 11-18)

The operating expenses section indicates that expenses for salaries and benefits, food, and supplies increased by 3.1 percent, 3.9 percent, and 2.3 percent, respectively. Other expenses decreased by 3.6 percent. However, the total operating expenses increased by $25,112, or 3.2 percent, over the budgeted amount. In addition, cash receipts are directly attributed to the improvement in cafeteria meals. At this point, the precise cost increases cannot be readily ascertained because of the fluctuation in the number of other meals served. When cash receipts from other nonpatient activities are applied against total operating expenses, the net dietary department expenses are $22,018, or 4.6 percent, over the budget.

4. Statistical Indicator/Cost Per Meal (lines 9-27)

The statistical indicator section details the operating expenses per meal for salary and benefits, food, supply, other expenses, and cash receipts. The net cost per meal is $1.28; this is 6.7 percent over the budgeted cost per meal of $1.20. The increase in operating expenses is further reflected in the net cost per patient day of $6.27, which is 7.4 percent over the budgeted amount of $5.84.

5. Productivity Indicators (lines 28-31)

A review of the productivity indicators shows that the food service department produced and served 5.39 meals per paid hour and 4.74 meals per worked hour, which are 4.3 percent and 4.2 percent, respectively, below the budgeted performance target. However, the number of meals served per patient day increased by 1.2 percent.

In summary, the financial operating data show the current expenditure of resources to provide meals for patient and nonpatient activities and also indicate how these expenditures compare with the budgeted resources and the projected productivity standards. The financial review of the operating data highlighted the variances from the fixed budget in spite of fluctuating volume. However, this is a cursory review; the food service administrator requires an in-depth financial analysis in order to ascertain the strength and weakness of the activity.

Evaluation of Financial Operating Data with Adjusted Budget

In order to evaluate the performance of the food service department, the budget is adjusted to reflect the projected cost at the current (actual) level of patient days and the number of patient and nonpatient meals served. To accomplish this evaluation, the budgeted patient days and total meals served are adjusted to correspond with the actual level. For example, table 1, lines 2 and 10 in the "actual" column show 80,350 patient days and 395,155 total meals served. These two important volume indicators are recorded in table 2, next page, under "revised budget." To determine the budgeted resources required to furnish the services listed under operating expenses, the revised budget column is adjusted in this manner:

Operating Expenses	Meals Served		Budget Unit Cost, $		Revised Budget, $
12. Salary and benefit expenses	395,155	×	0.86	=	339,833
13. Food expenses	395,155	×	0.87	=	343,785
14. Supply expenses	395,155	×	0.16	=	63,225
15. Other expenses	395,155	×	0.05	=	19,758
16. Total operating expenses					766,601
17. Less cash receipts	(395,155)	×	0.74	=	(292,415)
18. Net dietary expenses					474,186
26. Net cost per meal	$474,186 ÷ 395,155 = $1.20				
27. Net cost per patient day	$474,186 ÷ 80,350 = $5.90				

Table 2. Operating Statement and Revised Budget

Activity	Annual Total Actual	Annual Total Revised Budget	Variance	Percentage Variance	Cash Receipts Variance Applied on Basis of Percentage Variance	Adjusted Variance
2. Patient days	80,350	80,350	0			
10. Total meals	395,155	395,155	0			
11. **Operating Expenses**						
12. Salary and benefit expenses	$355,000	$339,833	+$15,167	+4.5%	40%	$3,184	$11,983
13. Food expenses	$362,750	$343,785	+$18,965	+5.5%	50%	$3,980	$14,985
14. Supply expenses	$ 66,250	$ 63,225	+$ 3,025	+4.8%	8%	$ 637	$ 2,388
15. Other expenses	$ 20,500	$ 19,758	+$ 742	+3.7%	2%	$ 159	$ 583
16. Total operating expenses	$804,500	$766,601	+$37,899	+4.9%	100%	$7,960	$29,939
17. Less cash receipts	($300,375)	($292,415)	+$ 7,960	+2.7%			
18. Net dietary expenses	$504,125	$474,186	+$29,939	+6.3%			
26. Net cost per meal	$ 1.28	$ 1.20	+$ 0.08	+6.7%			
27. Net cost per patient day	$ 6.27	$ 5.90	+$ 0.37	+6.3%			
28. **Productivity Indicators**						
29. Meals per hour—paid	5.39	5.63	− 0.24	−4.3%			
30. Meals per hour—worked	4.74	4.95	− 0.21	−4.2%			
31. Meals per patient day	4.92	4.86	− 0.06	+1.2%			
Hours—paid	73,313	70,187	+ 3,126	+4.4%			
Hours—worked	83,366	79,829	+ 3,537	+4.4%			

The revised budget amounts are clearly recorded in table 2. At this point, the revised budget and the actual expenditure are on the same basis, making the comparison more meaningful to the decision maker. The variance column shows that in each expense category, the actual expenditure exceeded the budgeted resources, as outlined below:

	Variance $	Variance %
16. Total operating expenses	+37,899	+4.9
17. Less cash receipts	+ 7,960	+2.7
18. Net dietary expenses	+29,939	+6.3
26. Net cost per meal	+0.08	+6.7
27. Net cost per patient day	+0.37	+6.3

The variance of $0.37, or 6.3 percent, in the net cost per patient day is significant. In addition, a review of these productivity indicators reinforces the fact that additional labor hours were used to produce a lower number of meals than that stated in the budget.

	Actual	Revised Budget	Variance, %
29. Meals per hour—paid	5.39	5.63	−4.3
30. Meals per hour—worked	4.74	4.95	−4.2

It is now clear that food service operating costs have risen above the authorized amounts and that the food service department has experienced a decrease in productivity in spite of a decline in the total number of meals served. The food service administrator will have to further investigate the reason for operating cost increases and prepare a corrective plan of action. To assist the food service administrator in identifying the operating cost increases, the following computation is made, again using table 2:

	Variance, $	Percentage Variance	Cash Receipts Variance Applied on Basis of % Variance, $	Adjusted Variance, $
12. Salary and benefit expenses	+15,167	40	3,184	11,983
13. Food expenses	+18,965	50	3,980	14,985
14. Supply expenses	+ 3,025	8	637	2,388
15. Other expenses	+ 742	2	159	583
16. Total operating expenses	+37,899	100	7,960	29,939
17. Less cash receipts	+ 7,960			
18. Net dietary expenses	29,939			

Using this method of computation, variances occurred in the following operating expenses: salary and benefit expenses, food expenses, supply expenses, and other expenses. In the next paragraphs, these areas of concern will be investigated further to ascertain the causes for these significant increases. Simultaneously, a general review of the important elements and features of each account will be discussed and recommendations will be made to improve this situation.

Review of Operating Procedures, Standards, and Expenses

A detailed review of the food service operating procedures, standards, and expenses covers the following major areas: food and supply costs, labor costs, other expenses, and nonpatient cash receipts.

Food and Supply Costs

To properly investigate the reason for the $14,985 adjusted variance in food costs and the $2,388 adjusted variance in supply costs shown in table 2, a review of the following activities needs to be completed.

Physical inventory

Compare the total inventory with that of previous months to ensure that variances are explainable. If there is a large difference in inventory totals, ascertain the composition of this difference. Check the quantities of the 30 major items and extend the cost. Verify the extension on all items in inventory.

Recording of invoices

Compare the purchase orders with the recording of invoices to ensure that all invoices are received, verified, recorded, and forwarded for payment. When goods are received without an invoice, the receiving copy of the purchase order should be priced and extended, and the total amount of the purchase should be accrued prior to the closing of the accounting period. The accrued amounts will be reversed upon receipt of an appropriate invoice.

Payment of invoices

Verify all paid invoices for an authorized signature. Compare the amount of paid invoices with the corresponding receiving reports for proper amounts and accuracy.

Receiving and storage procedures

Audit the receiving procedures for compliance with established standards of practice such as weighing goods, verifying quality, and counting items. This information is recorded on invoice and/or receiving reports. In addition, review the storage procedures for fresh and frozen foods, canned foods, and supplies. Proper receiving and storage procedures assist in maintaining the quality of the product and minimizing spoilage or waste.

Specifications and use of products

Investigate the use of the major products for proper specifications. The ideal situation is to provide the right product for the right recipe.

Production sheets or requisitions

Production sheets or requisitions are an important instrument of accountability. A production sheet shows the quantity of food ordered, the number of servings, the forecast amount, the actual number of portions served, and other remarks. A requisition serves as evidence of the quantity and description of the product received. Examining these records may verify the accuracy of forecasting and the number of portions served, and this, in turn, may facilitate narrowing the causes for overproduction or underproduction of foods.

Record of special events and menus

A careful review of the special events record may indicate the need for improved menu planning, pricing, and staffing requirements.

Food and supply index work sheets

An examination of the food and supply index work sheets reveals the actual percentage of increase based on purchases made during the period under study. For example, table 3, Food Cost Index Work Sheet, below, indicates that the increase in food costs from July 1982 to May 1983 is 9.5 percent. The 9.5 percent figure should be compared with the budgeted percentage in order to determine the extent of the financial impact on the food cost per meal. Similarly, table 4, Supply Cost Index Work Sheet, page 8, indicates that the increase in supply expenses from July 1982 to May 1983 is 18.2 percent. Again, the difference between 18.2 percent and the budgeted percentage, multiplied by the number of meals served, represents what the variance should be.

Menu

Studying the menu provides an insight into the type of food offered, the frequency, the cost, and the method of preparation. Preparing an attractive menu at a moderate cost requires the food service administrator to maintain a direct link between market prices and supply trends of meat, poultry, fish, canned goods, and vegetables.

These operating audit approaches may assist the food service administrator in understanding the impact of food costs on the financial statement. Furthermore, this type of audit provides the food service administrator with an opportunity to ascertain the flexibility of the menu and the degree of compliance with established operating standards and procedures.

In summary, an effective cost control system requires the development and implementation of policies and techniques that will minimize cost at every level of the operation.

Labor Cost

Salary and benefit expenses showed a significant increase of $11,983 over the budgeted amount. This increase in operating cost requires a review of labor activities, as outlined below, in order to ascertain the causes and, ultimately, ways to ameliorate the situation.

Table 3. Food Cost Index Work Sheet

May 1983
(Month, Year)

Food Expense	Baseline Value for July, 1982, $ (Month, Year)	Current Value, $	Weight per Category, %	Change per Category, %	Food Cost Index
Meat, fish, and poultry	674	744	.46	+.1039	.0478
Fresh produce	111	118	.02	+.0631	.0013
Frozen vegetables	152	163	.04	+.0724	.0029
Groceries	1,034	1,125	.34	+.0880	.0299
Milk and dairy	232	254	.08	+.0948	.0076
Bakery	173	189	.06	+.0925	.0055
Total	2,376	2,593	100.0		.0950

Table 4. Supply Cost Index Work Sheet

May 1983
(Month, Year)

Supply Expense	Baseline Value for July, 1982, $ (Month, Year)	Current Value, $	Weight per Category, %	Change per Category, %	Supply Cost Index
Disposables	742	880	.54	.1860	.1004
Cleaning supplies	112	115	.09	.0268	.0024
China and silverware	18	22	.32	.2222	.0711
Other	136	157	.05	.1544	.0077
Total	1,008	1,174	100.0		.1816

Labor time report

The use of the Labor Time Report (figure 1, following this chapter) enables the food service administrator to monitor the utilization of labor hours and to compare it with the budgeted hours. The variance between total paid hours and budgeted hours, which is expressed in hours and percentages, reflects the degree of attention this matter should receive. The report captures important information on food service performance standards for both patient and nonpatient activities and on the activities per patient day of clinical dietitians, dietetic technicians, and certified assistants. Such information can assist the food service administrator in measuring department performance and determining appropriate changes in directing the department. Also, use of this report provides important and timely information on labor time expenditure and the attainment of productivity standards. The information that this report can provide on the number of meals served puts the food service administrator in an excellent position to monitor payroll expenses in a timely fashion.

Work schedule

Usually, a work schedule lists the food service worker's name, position, shift hours, and days off. Scheduling the activities of food service workers requires planning, thought, and skill in order to fully utilize their services. Moreover, other important elements of scheduling include adequately defining the function that needs to be accomplished as well as the level of skill, effort, and time required to complete a given task. Thus, scheduling requires an in-depth knowledge of a particular task and an individual worker's ability to perform that task.

Other important scheduling techniques require understanding the following factors:

■ Volume forecasts and negotiated labor union contracts seriously affect managerial flexibility in maintaining an effective cost control over payroll expenses. In an effort to reduce or contain costs, the food service administrator may wish to consider rescheduling activities or reassigning functions based on the availability of workers' skills and volume forecasts.
■ The use of part-time workers provides flexibility and better utilization of personnel resources.
■ The provision of appropriate training enhances the workers' skills and motivates them to provide high-quality performance.
■ The effective food service administrator evaluates the productive use of workers during slow work activities. Advance production work may be scheduled, such as preparation of vegetables and juices, portioning, and so forth, during these slow periods in order to reduce labor costs.

- The menu should be evaluated to determine its effectiveness in offering a reasonable variety at an acceptable cost that makes efficient use of the workers' skills.
- The use of prepared foods in selective areas of the menu may prove beneficial.
- A substantial improvement in labor costs may result from the use of labor-saving equipment and devices. In the long-term, the investment in labor-saving equipment will be an effective way of reducing or containing cost. Some food service administrators have been able to improve the design and equipment layout of their food service department by relocating or consolidating such functions as warewashing, food production, and patient meal assembly line.

Finally, examining and reviewing work schedules and assigned tasks, rescheduling activities, volume forecasting, training and motivation, productivity standards, menu construction, use of ready foods, sick leave usage patterns, workers' skills, and labor saving equipment provide the food service administrator with opportunities to make informed decisions to reduce or contain labor costs.

In referring to the case study, the productivity indicators in table 2, page 4, showed a decline of 4.3 percent in meals served per paid hour that also resulted in an expenditure of 3,126 paid hours over the budgeted amount. The 3,126 paid hours represents the equivalent of 1.5 full-time employees (FTE). Of course, the cause for this apparent increase of 1.5 FTE is the decline in patient days and total meals served. With this information, the food service administrator can make an informed decision about the staffing levels in general and the reduction of 1.5 FTE in particular.

Other Expenses

To examine the adjusted variance of $583, the actual expenses should be compared to the budget and the significant difference should be identified. The general nature of these expense amounts is considered to be noncontrollable because there is no relationship between the number of meals served and such expenses as depreciation, insurance, dues, and subscriptions. These are fixed payments, or expenses, that are made periodically, regardless of the level of activity.

Nonpatient Cash Receipts

The following information can be derived from tables 1 and 2, pages 2 and 4:

	Annual Total Actual	Annual Total Budget	Variance
17. Cash receipts	$(300,375)	$(292,415)	+$ 7,960
6. Cafeteria meals	124,300	122,925	+ 1,375
8. Special functions	26,225	27,000	− 775
Total	150,525	149,925	+ 600
Average meal price	$ 1.9955	$ 1.9504	+$0.0451

It is obvious that cash receipts exceeded the budget by $7,960 for two reasons, namely the increase of 600 meals served and the increase of $0.0451 in the average meal price.

The increase in cash receipts needs to be further examined. An analysis of the $7,960 variance over the budget showed that the following factors contributed:

- Price: 150,525 meals served × $0.0451 price differential = $6,789
  (Average meal price: $1.9955 − $1.9504 = $0.0451)
- Volume: 600 meals served × $1.9504 = $1,171
  Total variance $7,960

It is clear that the amount of $6,789 resulted from an increase in the average selling price of meals in the cafeteria or at special functions. The effective food service administrator is able to determine precisely where these increases took place. On the other hand, the impact of the volume resulted in an increase of $1,171, which is minimal. Moreover, the meal composition was slightly altered as a result of the decrease in the actual patient meals and a corresponding increase in the actual nonpatient meals. These changes are outlined below:

4. Meal Count	Actual	Percentage	Budget	Percentage
5. Patient meals	224,980	56.9	231,000	57.6
6. Cafeteria meals	124,300	31.5	122,925	30.7
7. Stipend meals	19,650	5.0	19,950	5.0
8. Special function	26,225	6.6	27,000	6.7
10. Total meals	395,155	100	400,875	100

It is evident that patient meals declined by 0.7 percent (56.9 percent − 57.6 percent) and nonpatient meals increased by the same percentage (cafeteria 31.5 percent + special function 6.6 percent − cafeteria 30.7 percent + special function 6.7 percent). This shift may necessitate a reassignment of personnel from patient to nonpatient activities in order to maintain appropriate efficiency and balance.

The next process should involve the study of the food cost increases and the nonpatient menu pricing structure to verify the relationship between selling prices and food costs. The result of the menu study will indicate whether an increase in menu prices is appropriate.

Decision Making and Control

This case study indicates that patient days and meals have suffered a noticeable decrease, whereas operating costs such as food expenses, supply expenses, labor expenses, and other expenses increased significantly. In view of this formidable challenge, the food service administrator must make decisions to bring the food service department within the budgetary framework. To improve the operating costs, the following corrective actions should be taken:

- Reduce food costs
- Review menu
- Reduce labor by 1.5 FTEs and reassign staff to nonpatient activities
- Reduce other expenses

Moreover, nonpatient revenue and the number of meals increased significantly to warrant reviews of:

- Selling prices
- Menus
- Assignment of labor, workloads, tasks, and volume
- Supply expenses
- Other expenses

A further, more precise cost determination and allocation may be made if patient and nonpatient accounting functions are maintained separately, as suggested in the *Preparation of a Hospital Food Service Department Budget.*[1]

Note

[1] American Society for Hospital Food Service Administrators of the American Hospital Association. *Preparation of a Hospital Food Service Department Budget.* Chicago: AHA, 1978.

Bibliography

American Hospital Association. *Preparation of a Hospital Food Service Department Budget.* Chicago: AHA, 1978.

Atkinson, Alta B., and Blair, Eulalia C. *Volume Feeding Menu Selector.* New York: Cahners Publishing Company, Inc., 1971.

Berman, Howard J., and Weeks, Lewis E. *The Financial Management of Hospitals.* 5th ed. Ann Arbor, MI: Health Administration Press, 1981.

Cleverley, William O. One step further: the multivariable flexible budget system. *Hospital Financial Management.* 6:44, Apr. 1976.

Doyle, Stephen X., and Shapiro, Benson P. What counts most in motivating your sales force. *Harvard Business Review.* 58:133, May-June 1980.

Holder, W.W., and Wilhaurs, J. Better cost control with flexible budgets and variance analysis. *Hospital Financial Management.* 6:20, Jan. 1976.

Keiser, Ralph J., and Kallio, Elmer. *Controlling and Analyzing Costs in Food Service Operations.* New York City: John Wiley & Sons, Inc., 1974.

Kretschman, Carl G. Know how to analyze costs in evaluating savings projects. *Hospitals.* 50:69, Sept. 16, 1976.

Levinson, Charles. *Food and Beverage Operation.* Englewood Cliffs, NJ: Prentice-Hall, Inc., 1976.

Levitt, Theodore. Marketing success through differentiation—of anything. *Harvard Business Review* 58:83. Jan.-Feb. 1980.

Sasser Jr., W. Earl, and Leonard, Frank S. Let first-level supervisors do their job. *Harvard Business Review.* 58:113, Mar.-Apr. 1980.

Solomon, Kenneth I., and Katz, Norman. *Profitable Restaurant Management,* 2nd ed. Englewood Cliffs, NJ: Prentice-Hall, Inc., 1981.

U.S. General Accounting Office. *Study of Purchasing and Materials Management Functions in Private Hospitals.* Parts 1 and 2 (PSAD-79-58A and PSAD-79-58B). Washington, DC: U.S. General Accounting Office, 1979.

U.S. General Accounting Office. Report to the chairman, subcommittee on health, committee on finance, U.S. Senate. (HRD-80-35). Washington, DC: U.S. General Accounting Office, 1980.

Wenzel, Sr., George H. *Blueprints for Restaurant Success.* Austin, TX: George H. Wenzel Sr., 1973.

West, Bessie B., and others. *Food Service in Institutions.* 5th ed. New York City: John Wiley & Sons, Inc., 1977.

Figure 1. Sample Form for Labor Time Report

Labor Time Report

Cost center _____   Pay period ending _____

	Current	Year to Date
1. List employee hours as shown on time card		
Worked hours	_____	_____
Paid sick leave hours	_____	_____
Paid vacation hours	_____	_____
Paid holiday hours	_____	_____
Overtime hours	_____	_____
Total Paid Hours	_____	_____
Total Budgeted Hours	_____	_____
Variance	_____	_____
2. Calculate		
a. Meals per paid hour		
Actual	_____	_____
Budgeted	_____	_____
Variance	_____	_____
b. Clinical dietitians/technicians hours per patient day		
Actual	_____	_____
Budgeted	_____	_____
Variance	_____	_____
c. Number of cafeteria customers per paid hour		
Actual	_____	_____
Budgeted	_____	_____
Variance	_____	_____

3. Justify variance _____

4. Explain corrective action to be taken _____

5. List employee's name and paid hours

Vacation		Sick Leave		Holiday	
Name	Hours	Name	Hours	Name	Hours
_____	_____	_____	_____	_____	_____
_____	_____	_____	_____	_____	_____
Total Paid Hours _____		_____		_____	

Signature _____   Date _____

Budgetary Control Process

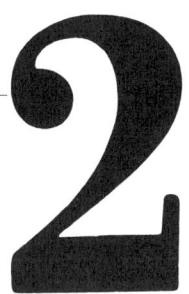

Chapter 2

The familiar refrains "I have a personnel problem, I need help" or "I just can't take on any additional duties without a few new bodies" point out that something is wrong in the area of staffing that cannot be ignored. The solution, in this case, appears obvious: hire more staff. But, more often than not, careful examination of the problem suggests that the solution is a more efficient utilization of present employees or a better distribution of work, not more people.

To deal effectively with this situation, food service administrators need a budgetary approach that clarifies objectives, specifies staffing levels, and provides a myriad of choices for the administration of the department. One such approach is known as project budgeting.

The project budgeting system provides a number of benefits to the food service department. It gives attention to the planning and controlling of activities. It enables the food service administrator to examine and analyze in depth the objectives, costs, and benefits of each level of expenditure for personnel and other resources. It forces hospital administration to analyze and decide on the discretionary cost areas. It reevaluates the priorities of the tasks and the performance of the activities. Moreover, during the project budgeting process, the food service administrator is provided with an opportunity to prepare and evaluate a number of contingency plans for the department. This process tends to develop capable managers who can cope with the challenges of managing hospital food services.

It is generally agreed that the proper design and use of the budget process is one of the most effective management tools because it does the following:

- States goals and objectives in a quantifiable manner
- Serves as a communication and commitment device for management
- Acts as a measurement tool and feedback for corrective action
- Points out deficiencies
- Forecasts when shortages might occur

Given the current emphasis on voluntary cost containment efforts and on managing with limited resources, better budgeting techniques are becoming more important to food service administrators. One tool is the project budgeting process, by which each activity must justify its budget request and no level of expenditure may be taken for granted.

The concept of project budgeting is gaining attention in view of the various hospital cost containment proposals, pending legislation, and government fiscal policies designed to substantially reduce health care expenditures and to closely monitor the level of health care being provided to Medicare and Medicaid patients.

However, the predominant budgetary practice today is still some form of incremental budgeting whereby the level of revenues and expenditures is projected for various levels of operations. Thus, applying the incremental approach to the budgeting process means that attention is directed to the changes that occur between the existing state and the proposed state. This process accepts the existing base and examines in detail only the increments that extend the current budgeting program into the future. The incremental procedure results in a continually upward-sloping expenditure line containing few declines or breaks.

Definition of Project Budgeting

Compared with this common practice of incremental budgeting, project budgeting differs markedly in structure, philosophy, and operation. Project budgeting is an organized process whereby resources are systematically assigned priorities and allocated according to anticipated outcomes. Each activity is identified as a decision package that is analyzed, evaluated, and ranked in order of its importance. This process involves all levels of management in the preparation of budgets.

A decision package is a form used to describe the resources required for each departmental activity to accomplish its stated objectives. A separate decision package is prepared for each level of service. It is customary to have at least three levels of service (minimum, current, and highest) for each departmental activity. As an example, figure 2A-P, following this chapter, outlines the required resources necessary to meet the objectives stated for the management of a food service department at the different levels of effort.

Methodology of Project Budgeting System

The project budgeting system has three main steps:

1. Describe each discrete activity on three levels of effort: minimum, current, and highest
2. Evaluate and rank all levels of effort or service
3. Allocate resources accordingly

To facilitate the review of the three incremental levels of effort, a decision package form is developed and used to capture the relevant data for meeting the specific objectives of each level of activity. The department head is required to furnish this information as follows:

1. Prepare objectives and performance standards
2. Prepare decision packages
3. Determine the cost for meeting objectives at the various levels of effort and effectiveness
4. Recommend priorities for all activities

In the next step, the hospital administrator evaluates the recommended priorities by:

1. Reviewing the recommended activities
2. Initiating desired changes to the priorities
3. Allocating resources to appropriate hospital departments for the fiscal year

Activity Levels for Decision Package

Typically, the first level of supervision in the hospital is responsible for preparing the decision package. To meet the departmental objectives at various levels of effort and effectiveness, the following guidelines are provided:

1. **Minimum** level of effort must be below current budget level of staffing and expenditure, for example 75 to 85 percent of the current budgeted amount, and at a critical level of effort, below which activity will cease to exist. [Activity at a critical level may be defined as activity that is (1) not completely achieving its objectives, (2) reducing the level of service, and (3) improving the level of efficiency.]
2. **Current** budgeted amount is classified as what could be achieved at the current level of efforts. In order to continue this level of activity in the following year, the budgeted amount needs to be adjusted for inflation.
3. **Highest** level of activity includes a budget for new programs or services to be performed.

Why are different levels of effort needed? On the surface, it appears that completing the decision package at various levels of effort and effectiveness involves excessive paperwork without clear benefit. However, there are two important reasons that justify the extra effort required. (1) There are limited funds available to any institution. Food service administrators believe that if only one level of effort is identified, some activities would be eliminated or arbitrarily reduced. In fact, the food service administrator will have an option between reducing the level of effort or eliminating the activity. In this situation, the food service administrator is in a position to make informed decisions on assigning resources according to established priorities. (2) Department heads and first-line supervisors are best equipped to identify and evaluate different levels of effort and effectiveness.

Ranking Process

After the initial development of the decision packages, the first-line supervisory personnel must become involved in the ranking process. For example, the food service administrator would be required to give a priority ranking to all decision packages submitted from unit supervisors who have already assigned their priority rankings. In practice, each decision package should be ranked in order of decreasing benefit to the institution. Essentially, supervisors should rank the decision packages that they have personally prepared, and food service administrators should rank the decision packages of all their subordinates.

Cutoff Point for Review

In an effort to review thoroughly each decision package, the hospital administrator will be faced with a monumental task of verifying priorities and rankings. Under these circumstances, it is doubtful that a thorough analysis could be completed. To substantially enhance this process, a hospital administrator may establish specific cutoff points for review. For example, each level of supervision could be required to review thoroughly only the lower 40 percent of the decision packages. The top-ranking packages would receive a cursory review.

Application of Project Budgeting System

The remainder of the chapter describes in detail how the project budgeting system can be applied to the hospital food service department. The major advantages of this specific budgetary approach to containing costs are delineated, and the benefit to the food service department is emphasized.

To begin planning for the application of the project budgeting system, important consideration has to be given to hospital goals and objectives for the period in question.

Statement of Hospital Objectives

The board of trustees and the hospital administration jointly formulate general goals and objectives for the direction of the institution. As an example, the following is a statement of goals for a university hospital:

- Provide patients with high-quality care by utilizing efficient and cost effective management systems and services, while emphasizing patient comfort and dignity
- Maintain an effective professional staff
- Develop new and innovative approaches for the organization and delivery of health care services
- Develop health care programs consistent with the educational mission of the university and the state and local health care needs
- Maintain a modern clinical environment for the education and training of health science students, staff members, and paramedical personnel
- Reduce the average length of stay and attempt to contain costs

Simultaneously, the hospital may issue specific forecasting guidelines such as the following:

Patient days	130,275
Length of stay	8.3
Admission	18,100
Salary increases	8%
Supply cost increases	8%
Food cost increases	10%
Clinic visits	205,800

Although it may be appropriate to have broad general goals for the hospital, goals for the food service department must be precise and consistent with the overall goals of the institution. To meet its overall goals, the food service department objectives may be stated as follows:

A. Maintain patient satisfaction level of 90 percent
B. Increase patient nutrition education program by 15 percent
C. Increase patient counseling and charting by 50 percent
D. Visit 95 percent of patients daily
E. Maintain average cost of meal at $4
F. Increase productivity rate to 3.9 meals per paid hour
G. Increase the dinner menu selection by five choices
H. Increase nonpatient revenue to $700,000

It is noteworthy that food service department objectives are stated in a quantifiable manner that both facilitates performance evaluation and provides a feedback system for management review and action.

At this point, the food service department receives organizational procedures for strategic and operational planning. These planning forecasts include hospital administration assumptions, policies, operating standards, and guidelines for expenditures, for example:

- Patient days will decrease by 3 percent
- Length of stay will decrease by 5 percent
- Admissions will not increase from previous budget year
- Seasonal patterns will continue as in previous 5 years
- Nonpatient feeding revenue will increase by 7 percent

Determination of the Organizational Relationships

In order to successfully implement the project budgeting concept, hospital administrators must have accurate knowledge about the organizational structure and relationships that exist in the hospital. The organizational structure must provide for an analysis of the tasks, jobs, or functions to be performed and an establishment of the relationships among departments. The tasks that will be necessary to accomplish the objectives must be (1) identified, (2) justified as being required, and (3) compatible and complementary to the other tasks to be performed. Related tasks must then be grouped together for greater efficiency in carrying them out and positioned within the organizational structure where they can be accomplished effectively. Furthermore, as the tasks in each group are interrelated, the most productive relationships among them must be established within the organizational structure.

Therefore, an essential ingredient in the implementation process of the project budgeting in the food service department is the identification of the organizational structure and the major activities providing services such as food production, meal service, nutrition education and patient nutritional service, purchasing and storage, nonpatient feeding, and administration of the food service department. The functional responsibility for the food service department is illustrated in figure 3, following this chapter. Figure 4, following this chapter, illustrates the interrelation of programs, functions, and resources. Once the identification of the food service department programs and functions has been accomplished, the second major task is to complete the decision packages.

Preparing the Decision Packages

The most important and challenging task for the food service administrator is to effectively prepare the decision packages, determine the cost for meeting objectives at the various levels of effort, and assign priorities for all activities. This task requires that the appropriate supervisors be involved in the planning of objectives for their respective food service function or program and in the development of the entire decision package. The decision package for each food service function or program includes documentation that details the following information:

- Description of the function
- Objective of the function
- Specific measures of performance
- Level of funding
- Projected costs for all resources required
- Benefit to be derived from funding
- Consequences to result from nonfunding
- Alternative ways of performing the same activity
- Ranking of the decision package

As an example, the food service department may have 16 decision packages, as illustrated in figures 2A through 2P, following this chapter. These decision packages indicate in detail the operational costs for varying levels of effort, propose alternative activity plans for achieving operational objectives, and determine resources necessary for alternative activity plans.

In other words, each package in this decision-package series represents an incremental level of expenditure for personnel, supplies, outside services, facilities, and equipment. Thus, each additional decision package comes closer to attaining or exceeding the stated objectives for the current level of service.

Actually, the different decision packages represent a range of options. Although the minimum level of effort, once it is identified, does not completely achieve the purpose of the function, it may, nevertheless, cover some of the more important elements. Thus, incremental levels of effort and funding, above the minimum level, are identified and ranked in order of importance. Also, at each level specific measures of performance are developed and stated. Therefore, project budgeting can be characterized as as process by which alternative approaches and alternative levels of activities are identified for attaining the objectives of a function.

Individual decision packages are prepared and completed for a discrete activity, at a specific level of effort and effectiveness, as illustrated in figure 2C.

Title: Food service department
Activity: Food production
Objective (as stated on page 16): A. Maintain patient satisfaction level of 90 percent; E. Maintain average cost of meal at $4; and F. Increase productivity rate to 3.9 meals (total department) per paid hour
Level 1 of 3: This entry indicates that there are three levels of effort. The first level is the minimum level required to maintain this activity without disruption in service.
Prepared: Signature of the preparer
Approved: Signature of hospital administrator
Date: Date of the decision package
Rank: Priority ranking assigned by director of food service, immediate supervisor, and hospital administrator

Purpose of activity: To provide food production for patient and nonpatient activities

Description of activity: The service volume is 738,280 total meals including nonpatient meals of 347,630 at level 1. This activity is responsible for forecasting meals, planning menus, requisitioning food and supplies, and preparing food.

Specific measures of performance: Three measures of performance are indicated: (1) cost per meal (production unit) = $0.89, (2) meals per paid hour = 13.15, and (3) patient satisfaction = 90 percent.

Advantage of retaining activity: Provides basic food production for patients and nonpatients

Consequences if activity is eliminated: Production service is essential for the hospital to maintain life, good nutrition, and satisfaction. (Note that at this level of funding, food production activity can attain only 70 percent of patient satisfaction because of the elimination of garnishes on meals.)

Alternative ways of performing work and costs: There are two options available: (1) purchase prepared foods at a cost of $700,000 or (2) hire a food service contractor to provide production services at an estimated cost of $675,000.

The required resources to support this activity are then identified.

Personnel: Number needed are estimated at 27 FTEs or 56,160 hours annually (27 FTE × 40 hours × 52 weeks)

Labor: Estimated at the current cost of $247,348 and forecast for budget year 1982-83 at an 8 percent increase (see hospital forecast guidelines) = $267,136

Food supply: Estimated at the current cost of $330,000 and forecast for budget year 1982-83 at 10 percent increase (see hospital forecast guidelines) = $363,000

Other expenses: Estimated at the current cost of $24,000 and forecast for budget year 1982-83 at 8 percent (see hospital forecast guidelines) = $25,920

Total cost: For this level at current prices, $601,348; for the budget year 1982-83, $656,056

The food production decision package at level 1 of 3 is now complete.

Ranking the Decision Packages

The next step in this process is for the director of food services to rank the decision packages in the order of decreasing benefit to the department (figure 5, following this chapter). This action identifies the benefits gained at each successive expenditure level and the disadvantages of not approving additional decision packages below a given expenditure level.

In reviewing the ranked food service department decision packages, the food service administrator has summarized expenditures at the following levels:

Level	Dollars	FTEs
Minimum	1,980,565	119
Current	2,135,616	133.5
Highest	2,376,616	134.5

The food service administrator and the hospital administration jointly have a wide range of selection among the various decision packages. To illustrate the variety of choices available for consideration, the following example outlines the options for only one unit (food production) in the food service department:

Food Production Budget Alternatives

Level	Dollars	FTEs
1	656,056	27
2 (1 and 2)	685,737	30
3 (1 and 3)	706,056	27 with menu choices
4 (1, 2 and 3)	735,737	30 with menu choices

In this example, the four levels of food production budget alternatives allow decisions to be made on the basis of priority ranking of packages as well as on the availability of resources. Also, each option has unique characteristics for accomplishing the stated objectives, specific measures of performance, the advantage of retaining the activity, an alternative way of performing the work and its cost, consequences if the activity is eliminated, and the estimated total cost for personnel, supplies, and other expenses.

Once the decision packages have been ranked, they are forwarded to the next higher organizational unit. At this level they are merged with other decision packages of comparable levels for review and reranking. This reranking would indicate the broader goals of the hospital as perceived at that organizational level.

Determination of Resource Allocation

The consolidated and ranked decision packages are reviewed and approved by the hospital administration. The final ranking then becomes the basis for resource allocation in determining the budget.

As the decision packages are consolidated and reranked, the perspectives and objectives are broadened. Generally, the consolidation and reranking of the decision packages are done by a committee that may consist of all managers whose packages are being ranked and a chairman selected from the next higher organizational level.

As the most essential decision packages will emerge toward the top of the final ranking and the least essential packages will gravitate toward the bottom, most of the scrutiny will be directed at the marginal packages—those that will be accepted or rejected on the basis of available resources.

A cutoff point may be used to facilitate the ranking of the competing packages at the various review levels. This cutoff point is an arbitrary percentage of the unit's current annual budget. Those packages ranked above the point are subjected to a cursory review. Packages ranked below this point are more vigorously examined for their relative contribution to the hospital's objectives.

When the approved budget is returned by the hospital administration, the food service administrator prepares an operating statement for each cost center and a consolidated operating statement for the entire department. During the budget year, the food service administrator prepares financial reports on the department performance (figure 6, following this chapter). These reports are reviewed jointly by the food service administrator and hospital administration to determine if reallocation of resources is needed.

Management Information System

In view of the high cost of personnel in hospitals, the hospital administrator needs to closely monitor the hiring of employees. To accomplish this objective, a position control system (figure 7, following this chapter) is established and properly supervised. The position control identifies vacant positions, cites funding levels from the approved budget, and eliminates the overhiring of personnel.

Furthermore, the use of a performance measure (figure 8, following this chapter) can greatly assist in objectively evaluating the performance of an activity or a department. This evaluative instrument, can facilitate the identification of both strong and weak areas of a department.

Benefits and Limitations of Project Budgeting System

The primary incentive for management to adopt project budgeting is the attainment of the following benefits:

■ Identifies the necessary resources required to accomplish the desired outcome
■ Highlights duplication of efforts among departments

■ Focuses on dollars needed for programs rather than on percent of change from previous budget year
■ Specifies priorities within and among departments and divisions
■ Allows comparisons of priorities across organizational lines
■ Facilitates performance audit to determine the degree of accomplishment of objectives

Ultimately, the benefits of the project budgeting system may be summarized as follows:

1. Planning and controlling activities

■ Activities are identified, evaluated, and justified
■ Resources are allocated on a systematic basis
■ Priorities proposed by lower management levels are approved by top management

2. Evaluating the results of activities

■ The manager is measured against objectives, performance, and benefits, as identified in decision packages
■ Poorly managed activities are readily identified

3. Developing human skills and interpersonal relationships

■ Thought processes for planning, operational control, efficiency, and cost effectiveness are developed in managers
■ Higher level of commitment is fostered

There are a number of limitations to the project budgeting process. Critics point out that it not only creates a large amount of paperwork, but also consumes time and valuable resources. In addition, the cost of implementing such a system is excessive. Critics contend that organizational politics dilute the strength and effectiveness of the system. However, in the final analysis, the success or failure of the project budgeting system is contingent on the sincere commitment of all levels of management in the health care institution.

Bibliography

American Society for Hospital Food Service Administrators of the American Hospital Association. *Preparation of a Hospital Food Service Department Budget.* Chicago: AHA, 1978.

Berman, Howard J., and Weeks, Lewis E. *The Financial Management of Hospitals.* 5th ed. Ann Arbor, MI: Health Administration Press, 1981.

Bowman, Richard M. Hospitals need new budgeting system. *Modern Healthcare.* 7:61, Aug. 1977.

Cleverley, William O. *Financial Management of Health Care Facilities.* Germantown, MD: Aspen Systems Corporation, 1976.

Goldman, Henry H. ZBB without paperwork. *Management Review.* 66:51, Oct. 1977.

Herkimer Jr., Allen G. *Understanding Hospital Financial Management.* Germantown, MD: Aspen Systems Corporation, 1978.

Pyhrr, Peter A. *Zero Base Budgeting: A Practical Tool for Evaluating Expenses.* (Systems and Controls for Financial Management Series). New York City: Wiley Interscience, 1973.

Suver, James D., and Brown, Ray. Where does zero base budgeting work? *Harvard Business Review.* 55:76, Nov.-Dec. 1977.

Suver, James D., and Neumann, Bruce R. Zero base budgeting. *Hospital and Health Services Administration.* 24:42, Spring 1979.

Figure 2A. Decision Package

Department Food Service	Objective No. All	Prepared		Date May 1982	
Activity Management	Level 1 of: 2 Minimum	Approved		Rank	
Purpose of Activity Direct and evaluate the departmental activities. Coordinate activities between and among departments. Provide secretarial help.			Resources Required	Current Year	Budget Year 82-83
			Personnel	3 FTEs 6,240 hours	3 FTEs 6,240 hours
Description of Activity Plan, organize, direct, and evaluate the activities of the Food Service Department.			Labor	$65,650	$70,902
			Supplies	4,500	4,860

Specific Measures of Performance
1. Patient satisfaction = 90% 4. Visit 95% of patients daily
2. Increase nutrition programs to 15 5. Cost per meal = $4.00
3. Increase counseling and 6. Meals per paid hour = 3.9
   charting to 50% 7. Increase dinner selection
                              by 5 choices
			Other	3,200	3,456

			Total	$73,350	$79,218

Advantage of Retaining Activity
Maintain leadership, control, and accountability over the entire Food Service Department.

Consequences if Activity is Eliminated
Loss of control and accountability over the food service functions. This staffing will cause a decrease of one-third of the secretarial work.

Alternative Ways of Performing Work and Costs
Hire an outside food service contractor at a cost of $120,000.

Figure 2B. Decision Package

Department Food Service	Objective No. E	Prepared		Date May 1982	
Activity Purchasing and storage	Level 1 of: 2 Minimum	Approved		Rank	
Purpose of Activity To purchase and store food and dietary supplies.			Resources Required	Current Year	Budget Year 82-83
			Personnel	1.0 FTE 2,080 hours	1.0 FTE 2,080 hours
Description of Activity Write specifications for products and service. Obtain prices and write purchase orders. Receive and store purchased products.			Labor	$11,000	$11,880
			Supplies	350	378
Specific Measures of Performance 1. 10 purchase orders per 4 hours 2. Process 15 requisitions per 4 hours			Other	70	76
			Total	$11,420	$12,334

Advantage of Retaining Activity
To maintain control and accountability over purchases and storage of food and dietary supplies.

Consequences if Activity is Eliminated
Loss of an essential part of control and accountability over purchase and storage of purchased supplies.

Alternative Ways of Performing Work and Costs
Hire an outside food service contractor at a cost of $16,000.

Figure 2C. Decision Package

Department Food Service	Objective No. A, E, F	Prepared		Date May 1982	
Activity Food production	Level 1 of: 3 Minimum	Approved		Rank	
Purpose of Activity Provide food production for patient and nonpatient activities.			Resources Required	Current Year	Budget Year 82-83
			Personnel	27 FTEs 56,160 hours	27 FTEs 56,160 hours
Description of Activity Volume: 738,280 meals (includes 347,630 nonpatient). Responsible for forecasting meals, planning menus, requisitioning food and supplies, and preparing food.			Labor	$247,348	$267,136
			Supplies	333,000	363,000
Specific Measures of Performance 1. Cost per meal = $0.89 3. Patient satisfaction = 90% 2. Meals per paid hour = 13.15			Other	24,000	25,920
			Total	$601,348	$656,056
Advantage of Retaining Activity Provide basic food production service.					
Consequences if Activity is Eliminated This service is essential for maintenance of life and good nutrition. This level provides patient satisfaction of only 70%. This level of effort does not fully meet objective A.					
Alternative Ways of Performing Work and Costs 1. Purchase ready foods at cost of $700,000. 2. Hire food service contractor at $675,000.					

Figure 2D. Decision Package

Department Food Service	Objective No. A, E, F	Prepared		Date May 1982	
Activity Meal service	Level 1 of: 3 Minimum	Approved		Rank	
Purpose of Activity Prepare, heat, and serve meals and nourishment to patients three times daily.			Resources Required	Current Year	Budget Year 82-83
			Personnel	48 FTEs 99,840 hours	48 FTEs 99,840 hours
Description of Activity Volume: 390,650 meals. Portion and assemble food for patients and nonpatients. Heat and serve meals and nourishment to patients. Warewashing for patient and nonpatient activities.			Labor	$446,685	$482,420
			Supplies	45,650	49,302
Specific Measures of Performance 1. Cost per meal = $1.41 3. Patient satisfaction = 90% 2. Meals per paid hour = 3.91			Other	18,476	19,954
			Total	$510,811	$551,676
Advantage of Retaining Activity Provide basic meal and nourishment service to patients.					
Consequences if Activity is Eliminated This service is essential for maintenance of life and good nutrition. Note: This level provides patient satisfaction of only 70%.					
Alternative Ways of Performing Work and Costs Hire an outside food service contractor at $625,000.					

Figure 2E. Decision Package

Department Food Service	Objective No. A, B, C, D	Prepared		Date May 1982	
Activity Nutrition service	Level 1 of: 3 Minimum	Approved		Rank	
Purpose of Activity Provide nutrition service and education to patients			Resources Required	Current Year	Budget Year 82-83
			Personnel	14 FTEs 29,120 hours	14 FTEs 29,120 hours
Description of Activity Volume: 130,275 patient days and 205,800 visits. Evaluate diets and menus. Counsel patient on good nutritional practices. Visit patient and evaluate their nutritional status. Chart in medical record. Provide educational programs.			Labor	$102,238	$110,417
			Supplies	6,315	6,820
Specific Measures of Performance 1. Dietitian paid hours per patient day = 0.22 2. Dietitian visit per patient day = 1.95	3. Dietitian counseling per patient day = .15 4. Cost per patient day = $0.92		Other	2,313	2,498
			Total	$110,866	$119,735

Advantage of Retaining Activity
Provide knowledge and education to patients and staff.

Consequences if Activity is Eliminated
This service is essential for maintenance of life and good nutrition.
Note: This level provides only 75% of visits and 35% of patient counseling and charting.

Alternative Ways of Performing Work and Costs
Hire an outside food service contractor at a cost of $125,000.

Figure 2F. Decision Package

Department Food Service	Objective No. H	Prepared		Date May 1982	
Activity Nonpatient feeding	Level 1 of: 3 Minimum	Approved		Rank	
Purpose of Activity Provide food service to employees and visitors.			Resources Required	Current Year	Budget Year 82-83
			Personnel	26 FTEs 54,080 hours	26 FTEs 54,080 hours
Description of Activity Volume: 330,250 meals; revenue = $700,030. Plan menus. Prepare and serve meals to employees and visitors. Serve special functions. Requisition food and supplies.			Labor	$240,613	$259,862
			Supplies	249,550	274,505
Specific Measures of Performance 1. Cash receipt per meal = $2.12 2. Cost per meal = $1.70	3. Meals per paid hour = 6.11		Other	25,166	27,179
			Total	$515,329	$561,546

Advantage of Retaining Activity
Maintain high morale among employees, and provide visitors with a convenient place to enjoy their meals.
Note: Soft ice cream is not provided.

Consequences if Activity is Eliminated
Employees and visitors morale will be low. Employees will take longer breaks to obtain their meals from outside the hospital.

Alternative Ways of Performing Work and Costs
Hire an outside food service contractor at a cost of $150,000.

Figure 2G. Decision Package

Department Food Service	Objective No. All	Prepared		Date May 1982	
Activity Management	Level 2 of: 2 Current	Approved		Rank	
Purpose of Activity			Resources Required	Current Year	Budget Year 82-83
			Personnel	1.0 FTE 2,080 hours	1.0 FTE 2,080 hours
Description of Activity			Labor	$8,500	$9,180
			Supplies		
Specific Measures of Performance			Other		
			Total	$8,500	$9,180

Advantage of Retaining Activity
This level of staffing ensures that secretarial work is provided to food service units on an as needed basis.

Consequences if Activity is Eliminated
The reduction in secretarial staffing may cause delays of up to three or four weeks in providing service to food service units.

Alternative Ways of Performing Work and Costs
There is no lower cost alternative available.

Figure 2H. Decision Package

Department Food Service	Objective No.	Prepared		Date May 1982	
Activity Purchasing and storage	Level 2 of: 2 Current	Approved		Rank	
Purpose of Activity			Resources Required	Current Year	Budget Year 82-83
			Personnel	0.5 FTE 1,040 hours	0.5 FTE 1,040 hours
Description of Activity			Labor	$4,020	$4,342
			Supplies		
Specific Measures of Performance			Other		
			Total	$4,020	$4,342

Advantage of Retaining Activity
This level of staffing provides for better control over receiving and issuing procedures.

Consequences if Activity is Eliminated
Loss of 20% of internal control over receiving and issuing procedures.

Alternative Ways of Performing Work and Costs
There is no lower cost alternative available.

Figure 2I. Decision Package

Department Food Service	Objective No. A, E, F	Prepared		Date May 1982	
Activity Food production	Level 2 of: 3 Current	Approved		Rank	
Purpose of Activity Provide food production for patient and nonpatient activities..			Resources Required	Current Year	Budget Year 82-83
			Personnel	3 FTEs 6,240 hours	3 FTEs 6,240 hours
Description of Activity Volume: 738,280 meals. Responsible for forecasting meals, planning menus, requisitioning food and supplies, and preparing food.			Labor	$27,482	$29,681
			Supplies		
Specific Measures of Performance Cost per meal = $0.93 Patient satisfaction = 90% Meals per paid hour = 11.83			Other		
			Total	$27,482	$29,681
Advantage of Retaining Activity Provide basic food production service. Note: Objectives will be achieved.					
Consequences if Activity is Eliminated Patient satisfaction level will be at 70%.					
Alternative Ways of Performing Work and Costs 1. Purchase ready foods at cost of $710,000. 2. Hire food service contractor at $685,000.					

Figure 2J. Decision Package

Department Food Service	Objective No. A, E, F	Prepared		Date May 1982	
Activity Meal service	Level 2 of: 3 Current	Approved		Rank	
Purpose of Activity			Resources Required	Current Year	Budget Year 82-83
			Personnel	6 FTEs 12,480 hours	6 FTEs 12,480 hours
Description of Activity Volume: 390,650 meals. Portion and assemble food for patients and nonpatients. Serve meals and nourishment. Warewashing.			Labor	$55,835	$60,302
			Supplies		
Specific Measures of Performance 1. Cost per meal = $1.57 3. Patient satisfaction = 90% 2. Meals per paid hours = 3.48			Other		
			Total	$55,835	$60,302
Advantage of Retaining Activity Provide adequate meal service to patients and nonpatients. Objectives will be completely achieved.					
Consequences if Activity is Eliminated Patient satisfaction level will be at 70%.					
Alternative Ways of Performing Work and Costs There is no lower cost alternative available.					

Figure 2K. Decision Package

Department	Objective No.	Prepared	Date
Food Service	A, B, C, D		May 1982
Activity	**Level 2 of: 3**	**Approved**	**Rank**
Nutrition service	Current		

	Resources Required	Current Year	Budget Year 82-83
Purpose of Activity	Personnel	2 FTEs 4,160 hours	2 FTEs 4,160 hours
Description of Activity Volume: 130,275 patient days; 205,800 visits	Labor	$14,605	$15,773
	Supplies		
Specific Measures of Performance 1. Dietitian's paid hours per patient day = 0.26 3. Dietitian's counseling per patient day = 0.20 2. Dietitian's visit per patient day = 2.00 4. Cost per patient day = $1.04	Other		
	Total	$14,605	$15,773

Advantage of Retaining Activity
Meet all the stated objectives.

Consequences if Activity is Eliminated
This level of staffing will provide 75% of visits and 35% of patient counseling and charting.

Alternative Ways of Performing Work and Costs
There is no lower cost alternative available.

Note: Recommend hiring two dietary technicians with two years specialized training.

Figure 2L. Decision Package

Department	Objective No.	Prepared	Date
Food Service	H		May 1982
Activity	**Level 2 of: 3**	**Approved**	**Rank**
Nonpatient feeding	Current		

	Resources Required	Current Year	Budget Year 82-83
Purpose of Activity	Personnel	2 FTEs 4,160 hours	2 FTEs 4,160 hours
Description of Activity Volume: 347,630 meals; revenue: $747,400.	Labor	$18,507	$19,988
	Supplies	8,450	9,295
Specific Measures of Performance 1. Cash receipt per meal = $2.15 3. Meals per paid hour = 6.0 2. Cost per meal = $1.72	Other	6,009	6,490
	Total	$32,966	$35,773

Advantage of Retaining Activity
This level of effort provides staffing for the soft ice cream station. Additional revenue pays for cost of labor and supplies.

Consequences if Activity is Eliminated
The requests for soft ice cream will not be fulfilled.

Alternative Ways of Performing Work and Costs
There is no lower cost alternative available.

Figure 2M. Decision Package

Department	Objective No.	Prepared		Date
Food Service	G			May 1982
Activity	Level 3 of: 3	Approved		Rank
Food production	Highest			

Purpose of Activity	Resources Required	Current Year	Budget Year 82-83
	Personnel		
Description of Activity	Labor		
	Supplies		$50,000
Specific Measures of Performance 1. Cost per meal = $1.00	Other		
	Total		$50,000

Advantage of Retaining Activity
Increase patient satisfaction and provide wider selection of modified diets.

Consequences if Activity is Eliminated
Continued complaints about limited selection for patients on modified diets.

Alternative Ways of Performing Work and Costs
There is no lower cost alternative available.

Figure 2N. Decision Package

Department	Objective No.	Prepared		Date
Food Service	New			May 1982
Activity	Level 3 of: 3	Approved		Rank
Meal service	Highest			

Purpose of Activity	Resources Required	Current Year	Budget Year 82-83
	Personnel		
Description of Activity Volume: 390,650 meals.	Labor		
	Supplies		
Specific Measures of Performance 1. Cost per meal = $1.69	Other		$50,000
	Total		$50,000

Advantage of Retaining Activity
To improve menu appearance.

Consequences if Activity is Eliminated
Occasional complaints and remarks about menu appearance.

Alternative Ways of Performing Work and Costs
Outside consultant fee may exceed $65,000 in expenditures.

Figure 2O. Decision Package

Department Food Service	Objective No. New	Prepared		Date May 1982	
Activity Nutrition service	Level 3 of: 3 Highest	Approved		Rank	
Purpose of Activity			Resources Required	Current Year	Budget Year 82-83
			Personnel		1 FTE 2,080 hours
Description of Activity Volume: 130,275 patient days; 205,800 visits.			Labor		$16,000
			Supplies		
Specific Measures of Performance 1. Dietitian's paid hour per patient day = 0.27 2. Cost per patient day = $1.16			Other		
			Total		$16,000

Advantage of Retaining Activity
Increase the Nutrition Clinic activity by 100%, and increase patient education.

Consequences if Activity is Eliminated
Continued remarks about the unavailability of dietitian for service at time of Medicine Clinic visit.

Alternative Ways of Performing Work and Costs
There is no lower cost alternative available.

Figure 2P. Decision Package

Department Food Service	Objective No. New	Prepared		Date May 1982	
Activity Nonpatient feeding	Level 3 of: 3	Approved		Rank	
Purpose of Activity			Resources Required	Current Year	Budget Year 82-83
			Personnel		
Description of Activity Volume: 347,630 meals; revenue: $747,400.			Labor		
			Supplies		
Specific Measures of Performance 1. Cost per meal = $2.08			Other		$125,000
			Total		$125,000

Advantage of Retaining Activity
Decorate cafeteria to enhance the dining atmosphere, increase revenue by 5%, and boost employee morale.

Consequences if Activity is Eliminated
Occasional comments about the dull appearance of dining room.

Alternative Ways of Performing Work and Costs
There is no lower cost alternative available.

Figure 3. Organizational Chart of Functional Responsibilities in a Food Service Department

- Board of Trustees
  - Administration
    - Assistant Administrator
    - Assistant Administrator
    - Assistant Administrator
      - Director, Food Service Department
        - Management
          - Food Production
            - Menu forecasting
            - Menu planning
            - Food preparation
            - Facility sanitation
          - Meal Service
            - Assembly of food and meal service
            - Distribution of meals
            - Washing
          - Nutrition Service
            - Counseling
            - Visitation
            - Charting
            - Education
          - Purchasing and Storage
            - Specification
            - Purchasing
            - Receiving
            - Storage
            - Distribution
          - Nonpatient Feeding, Cafeteria
            - Employees
            - Visitors
            - Special functions
      - Director, Department
      - Director, Department
      - Director, Department
      - Director, Department

Budgetary Control Process ■ 29

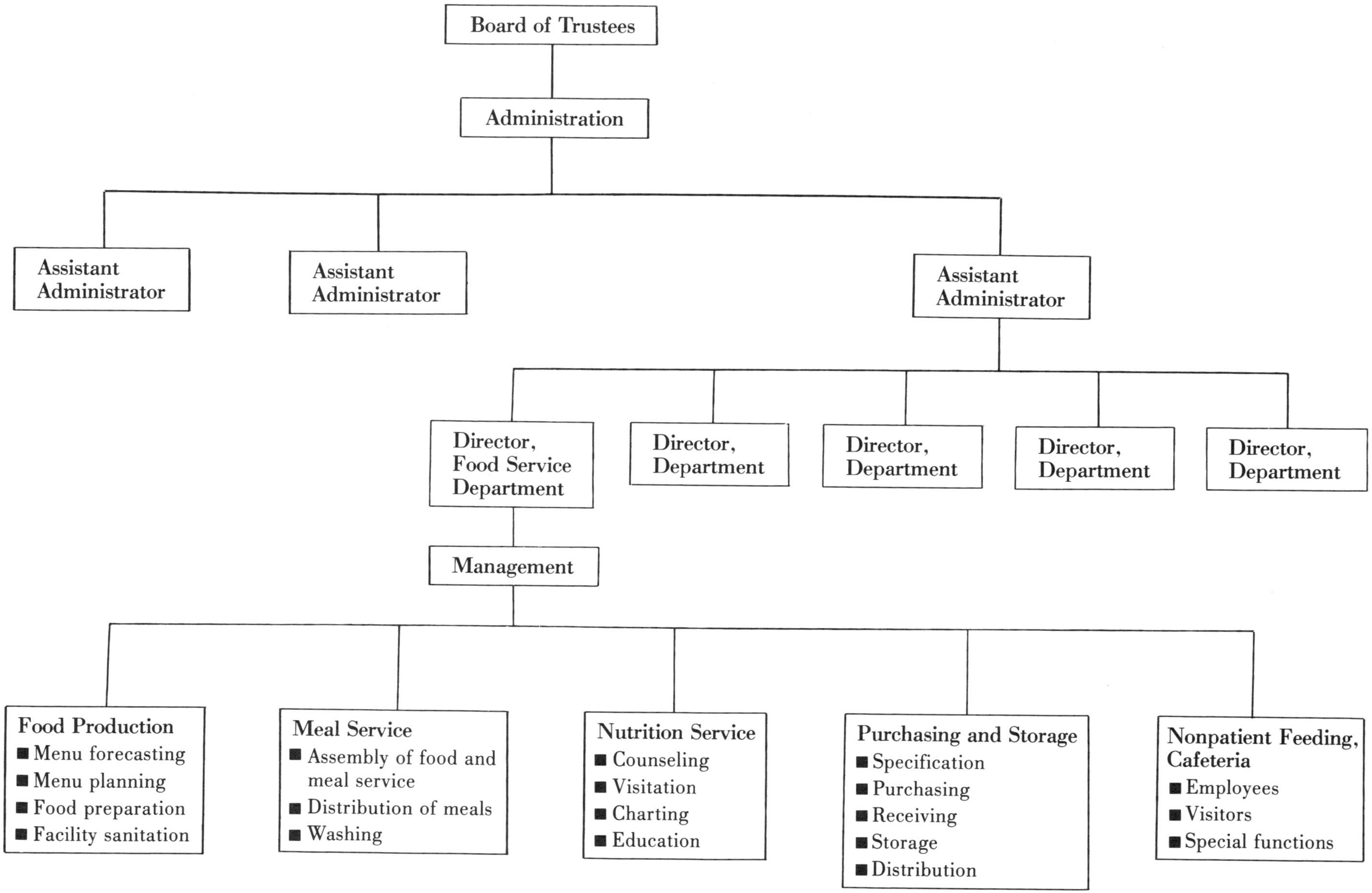

Figure 4. Food Service Department Activity

Programs	Functions	Resources
Food production	Menu forecasting	Management and supervision
■ General and modified meals	Menu planning	Employees
■ Nonpatient meals	Food preparation	Equipment
	Assembly of food and meal service	Facilities
Meal service	Distribution of meals	Supplies
	Counseling	Money
Nutrition education	Visitation	
■ Patient	Charting	
■ Public	Education	
	Specification	
Nutrition service	Purchasing	
■ Patient	Receiving	
	Storage	
Purchasing and storage	Distribution	
■ Patient	Nonpatient meal service	
■ Public	Washing	
	Facility sanitation	
Nonpatient feeding	Management	
■ Employees		
■ Visitors		
■ Special functions		

Figure 5. Example of Priority Ranking

Date: May 1982

Department	Division	Prepared	Page
Food Service		Approved	1 of 2

	Activity	Level		Current Year		Budget Year		Cumulative
Rank	Name and Description	No.	of No.	Personnel	$ (000)	Personnel	$ (000)	$ (000)
1	Management	1	2	3	73,350	3	79,218	79,218
2	Purchasing and storage	1	2	1	11,420	1	12,334	91,552
3	Food production	1	3	27	601,348	27	656,056	747,608
4	Meal service	1	3	48	510,811	48	551,676	1,299,284
5	Nutrition service	1	3	14	110,866	14	119,735	1,419,019
6	Nonpatient feeding	1	3	26	515,329	26	561,546	1,980,565
7	Management	2	2	1	8,500	1	9,180	1,989,745
8	Purchasing and storage	2	2	0.5	4,020	0.5	4,342	1,994,087
9	Food production	2	3	3	27,482	3	29,681	2,023,768
10	Meal service	2	3	6	55,835	6	60,302	2,084,070
11	Nutrition service	2	3	2	14,605	2	15,773	2,099,843
12	Nonpatient feeding	2	3	2	32,966	2	35,773	2,135,616
13	Food production	3	3	0	0	0	50,000	2,185,616
14	Meal service	3	3	0	0	0	50,000	2,235,616
15	Nutrition service	3	3	0	0	1	16,000	2,251,616
16	Nonpatient feeding	3	3	0	0	0	125,000	2,376,616
	Total			133.5	1,966,532	134.5	2,376,616	

Figure 6. Sample Form for Financial Reports

Explanation of and Comments on
Significant Budget Changes

Cost center _____   Name _____

Volume _____
_____

Revenue _____
_____

Personnel _____
_____

Expenses _____
_____

Capital expenditure _____
_____

Suggested Purchase Date	Description	Cost	Priority of Need
_____	_____	_____	_____
_____	_____	_____	_____

Priority of Need

A.	Urgent	Necessary to maintain the hospital's level of patient care
B.	Essential	Required to replace vital and necessary equipment worn out or out of order
C.	Economically desirable	Would improve current services or add new services
D.	Desirable	Would replace nonessential equipment

Figure 7. Sample Form for Position Control

Position Control

1. Request for Hiring

Request by _____ Date of request _____
(Name of department head or supervisor)

Classification of position
to be cleared for hiring _____

Location of position _____ Percent of full time _____
(Cost center number)   (Hours per week if less than 40)

Name, class, and position number
of terminating employee _____

Expected date
of termination _____ Number of hours accrued for vacation _____
(Last day worked)

Requested starting
date of replacement _____ Requested starting salary if higher than class minimum _____

2. Review and Approval by Administrative Council Member

Date reviewed and approved   Reviewed and approved by

_____   _____
                                          (Signature of council member)

3. Budget Office Verification of Position and Fund Availability

Position budgeted at   Position budget at _____
% requested _____   _____ % of full-time

Fund Availability

Verified by _____   Date of verification _____

Figure 8. Sample Form for Measuring Performance

Food Service Department
Patient Questionnaire

The food service department is interested in your comments about the meal service in the hospital. Your cooperation in completing this questionnaire will be most helpful and appreciated. Keep the completed form with your menu and a dietitian or a dietetic technician will pick it up. Thank you.

Date _____

1. Name _____ Room no. _____ Unit _____

2. Did a dietitian or a dietetic technician visit you? Yes _____ No _____

3. Are you on a modified diet?   Yes _____ No _____

   Name of diet _____

   If you are on a modified diet, has it been explained to you by a dietitian?   Yes _____ No _____

4. For each topic, check (X) the phrase that best describes your opinion of that aspect of food service. Please feel free to make any additional comments in the section below.

	Good	Fair	Poor	Comments
Meal appearance				
Quality of food				
Flavor of food				
Hot food temperature				
Cold food temperature				
Portion sizes				
Menu variety				

5. General comments _____

   _____

   _____

   _____

Capital Investment Analysis

Chapter 3

Capital investment analysis is one of the most important management tools in evaluating capital expenditure alternatives. The selection of the appropriate capital expenditure plan will have an impact on future operations and cash flow over an extended period of time regardless of volume fluctuations.

The involvement of the department administrator and the supervisors in identifying capital expenditure alternatives cannot be overemphasized. Departmental objectives stem primarily from programs and plans prepared and approved by the department administrator. Thus, the department administrator is in the most strategic position to identify the department's particular capital asset needs and give priority ranking to these needs.

One of the major responsibilities of all administrators is the efficient and effective allocation of scarce economic resources. This activity requires the knowledge and skill necessary to objectively evaluate a range of capital expenditure alternatives.

Capital Equipment Evaluation Program

There are a number of methods by which a health care institution can evaluate capital equipment requests. Health care institutions have gradually adopted procedures to review capital equipment requests, to rank them, and to efficiently allocate scarce economic resources. A capital equipment evaluation program usually includes the following:

■ **Classification by cost category.** A health care institution may establish a capital equipment evaluation program that includes all items valued at less than $200. Thus, for all items valued at more than $200, the administrator would be required to furnish detailed information, as shown in figure 9, following this chapter.

■ **Intended use.** The department requesting the purchase of particular equipment is required to provide a general description of the intended use, list the benefits, and suggest possible alternatives. Each request has to be given a priority ranking according to the needs of the department. Three levels of priority are defined as follows: (1) The *urgent* level of priority denotes that the particular piece of equipment is necessary to maintain patient care, (2) the *essential* level of priority indicates that the equipment is needed to replace worn-out or out-of-order equipment, and (3) the *desirable* level of priority applies to equipment that is required to improve current practice or is designed to be part of a new service.

■ **Financial evaluation.** The financial evaluation of a capital equipment request centers on the size of the investment, the revenue to be generated, the operating costs, and the amount of savings to be realized.

■ **Ranking of request.** Hospital administrators have the responsibility to determine both the amount of resources available for capital equipment purchases and a system for ranking requests based on these important factors: the merit of the request, the amount of initial investment, the amount of future cash inflows and/or outflows, and the cost of total lifetime investments.

■ **Acquiring approval.** The final step in the capital equipment evaluation program is the attainment of various approvals from the hospital administration, the hospital board, health planning councils, and other agencies.

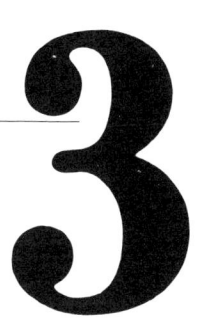

Financial Evaluation of Capital Investment Alternatives

There are five methods of capital investment evaluation being used in the health care field: the payback period, the average rate of return, the internal rate of return (or time-adjusted rate of return), the net present value, and life-cycle costing. Although the health care field in general has been reticent to use these methods of financial evaluation, there has been a noticeable increase in their use in recent years.

Payback Period

Payback period is defined as the length of time required for the cash proceeds from investment to equal the original investment cost. The formula is as follows: divide the cost of the investment by the annual cash flow; the answer is in number of years.

$$\frac{\text{Investment}}{\text{Annual operating savings (annual cash flow)}} = \text{Payback, in number of years}$$

For example: The purchase price of an electronic cash register is $5,000. It has a useful life of 10 years with no salvage value. The estimated operating savings is $800 per year, and money can be borrowed or invested at 8 percent or 16 percent. Depreciation is calculated at $500 per year. To evaluate this purchase under the payback technique, divide the purchase price by the estimated operating savings ($5,000 ÷ $800 = 6.25 years). It will take 6.25 years to pay the $5,000 for the cost of an electronic cash register based on the estimated operating savings of $800 per year.

The payback technique is one of the simplest and most frequently used methods for evaluating capital investments. However, it should be noted that the payback technique has certain shortcomings: it does not account for the cost of interest on the invested money; it does not include the life of the equipment; and it does not account for depreciation expenses when the financial investment is considered. This method is appropriate to use when the payback period is about a year or less.

Average Rate of Return

The average rate of return is defined as the average ratio of earnings to the book value of the investment. The formula is as follows: divide earnings by the book value of the investment, or subtract the depreciation from the operating savings and divide that figure by the investment.

$$\frac{\text{Earnings}}{\text{Book value}} = \text{Average rate of return}$$

or

$$\frac{\text{Operating savings} - \text{Depreciation}}{\text{Investment}} = \text{Average rate of return}$$

To evaluate the previous example (purchasing the electronic cash register) under the average rate of return technique, the appropriate figures are plugged into the formula:

$$\frac{\$800 - \$500}{\$5,000} = .06$$

This method of financial evaluation excludes the cost of interest on the investment and the life of the equipment.

Discounted Cash Flow

The concept of discounted cash flow recognizes that the use of money has a cost (interest) and assumes that a dollar today is worth more than a dollar five years from now. It is considered to be one of the best methods for long-range capital decisions because it weighs the time value of money and focuses on the cash inflows and cash outflows. In addition, the discounted cash flow has two variations to compute future worth of return: the internal rate of return (time-adjusted rate of return) and the net present value.

Internal Rate of Return

The internal rate of return (time-adjusted rate of return) is defined as the rate that will make cash inflows equal to cash outflows. The formula is as follows:

$$\text{For a particular period,} \quad \frac{\text{Investment}}{\text{Operating savings}} = \text{Present worth of \$1 per period}$$

Again, applying the internal rate of return technique to the example of the purchase of the electronic cash register, the formula works as follows:

$$\text{For 10 years,} \quad \frac{\$5,000}{\$800} = 6.25$$

As can be seen from table 5, next page, 6.25 for 10 years falls between 8 percent and 10 percent. In this example, the identification of the interest rate as being between 8 percent and 10 percent is adequate. To find the precise internal rate of return for the present value of inflows of 6.25, the following equation should be set up:

Interest Rates	Present Value of Inflows
8%	= 6.710
i	= 6.25
10%	= 6.145

Where: i indicates interest rate.
The difference in interest rate between 10 percent and 8 percent is 2 percent.
The difference in the present value of inflows between 6.710 and 6.145 is 0.565, and between 6.710 and 6.25 is 0.46.

$0.565 = 2\%$
$0.46 = i$
$$\frac{0.46 \times 2\%}{0.565} = 1.63\%$$

The precise internal rate of return is 8 percent + 1.63 percent = 9.63 percent. This percentage takes into account the investment, the operating savings, the life of equipment, and the interest rate. Table 6, page 39, shows a year-by-year analysis of the earnings of 9.63 percent on invested capital (electronic cash register, $5,000) and the amount of recovery of investment over 10 years. Thus, the investment of $5,000 with a net cash inflow of $500 per year for a period of 10 years yields 9.63 percent.

Table 5. Present Value of Ordinary Annuity of $1.00, Selected Values

Period, Years	8%	10%	16%	20%
1	0.928	0.909	0.862	0.833
2	1.783	1.736	1.605	1.528
3	2.577	2.487	2.246	2.106
4	3.312	3.170	2.798	2.589
5	3.993	3.791	3.274	2.991
6	4.623	4.355	3.685	3.326
7	5.206	4.868	4.039	3.605
8	5.747	5.335	4.344	3.837
9	6.247	5.759	4.607	4.031
10	6.710	6.145	4.833	4.192
11	7.139	6.495	5.029	4.327
12	7.536	6.814	5.197	4.439
13	7.904	7.103	5.342	4.533
14	8.244	7.387	5.468	4.611
15	8.559	7.606	5.575	4.675

Net Present Value

The net present value concept operates on the premise that cash inflows and/or outflows are discounted to the present time at a predetermined, or desired, rate of return. The formula is as follows:

Inflow × Present value of ordinary annuity of $1 − Investment = Net present value

Once again, take the example of the purchase of the electronic cash register at 8 percent interest and apply the net present value concept as follows:

$800 × 6.71 − $5,000 = +$368

The rate of 6.71 was taken from table 5, above, for a period of 10 years at an interest rate of 8 percent. The result is plus $368 (greater return over the life of the project than the initial investment), therefore the proposed capital project is desirable because its return exceeds the desired minimum. Table 7, page 39, shows the effect of the $800 net cash inflow discounted at 8 percent for each year over a period of 10 years.

Now, suppose you wish to purchase the electronic cash register for $5,000 with a 10-year life and a cash inflow of $800 per year, but you desire to obtain a rate of 16 percent. The calculation would be as follows:

Inflow × Present value of ordinary annuity of $1 − Investment = Net present value

or

$800 × 4.833 − $5,000 = −$1,134

The rate of 4.833 was taken from table 5, above, for a period of 10 years at an interest rate of 16 percent. Because the result is negative, the proposal is mathematically undesirable. Table 8, page 40, outlines the effect of the $800 net cash inflow, discounted at 16 percent, for each year over a period of 10 years.

Table 6. Earnings at 9.63 Percent on Invested Capital and Recovery of Investment in 10 Years

Year	Unrecovered Capital at Beginning of Year, $	Net Cash Inflow, $	Return at 9.635% on Unrecovered Capital, $	Amount of Capital Recovered, $
1	5,000	800	482	318
2	4,682	800	451	349
3	4,333	800	417	383
4	3,950	800	380	420
5	3,530	800	340	460
6	3,070	800	296	504
7	2,566	800	247	553
8	2,013	800	194	606
9	1,407	800	136	664
10	743	800	72	728
Total		8,000	3,015	4,985

The amount of capital recovered equals net cash inflow minus return on unrecovered capital: $4,985 = $8,000 − $3,015.

Calculation:

First year
Return of unrecovered capital: $5,000 × 0.0963 = $482
Amount of capital recovered: $800 − 482 = $318

Second year
Unrecovered capital at
  beginning of the year: $5,000 − 318 = $4,682
Return of unrecovered capital: $4,682 × 0.0963 = $451
Amount of capital recovered: $800 − 451 = $349

Table 7. Present Net Value with Cash Inflow Discounted at 8 Percent

Year	Present Value of $1.00 Discounted at 8%, $	Net Cash Inflow, $	Total Present Value, $
1	0.926	800	741
2	0.857	800	686
3	0.794	800	635
4	0.735	800	588
5	0.681	800	545
6	0.630	800	504
7	0.583	800	467
8	0.540	800	432
9	0.500	800	400
10	0.463	800	370

Total present value of future cash inflows   5,368
Less original investment   (5,000)
Total return on investment   368

Table 8. Present Net Value with Cash Inflow Discounted at 16 Percent

Year	Present Value of $1.00 Discounted at 16%, $	Net Cash Inflow, $	Total Present Value, $
1	0.862	800	690
2	0.743	800	594
3	0.641	800	513
4	0.552	800	442
5	0.476	800	381
6	0.410	800	328
7	0.354	800	283
8	0.305	800	244
9	0.263	800	210
10	0.227	800	181

Total present value of future cash inflows   3,866
Less original investment   (5,000)
Total return on investment   (1,134)

Life-Cycle Costing

The life-cycle costing method is defined as the process by which a capital expenditure is evaluated against alternatives by computing total costs over the anticipated life span of the asset or the program. Included are operating costs for personnel, materials and supplies, maintenance and operations, and allocated overhead. The investment and equipment costs as well as a factor for inflation and a discounted rate of return are determined for each individual capital investment.

Suppose a food service administrator is considering replacing the existing meal assembly line with a fully automated one. The administrator has received two alternative proposals for this project, which contained the following information:

Alternative A

Cost of equipment—$95,000 with the following estimated operating expenses occurring in the first year:

- Salary expenses of $8,500 with an estimated annual increase of 10 percent
- Supply expenses of $200 with an estimated annual increase of 12 percent
- Maintenance expenses of $1,500 with an estimated annual increase of 15 percent
- Allocated overhead of $2,000 with an estimated annual increase of 15 percent

It is expected that the meal assembly line will have a 10-year useful life.

Alternative B

Cost of equipment—$40,000 with the following estimated operating expenses occurring in the first year:

- Salary expenses of $11,200 with an estimated annual increase of 10 percent
- Supply expenses of $350 with an estimated annual increase of 12 percent
- Maintenance expenses of $2,500 with an estimated annual increase of 15 percent
- Allocated overhead of $2,000 with an estimated annual increase of 15 percent

It is expected that the meal assembly line will have a 10-year useful life. The food service administrator would like to obtain 14 percent on the invested money.

Table 9, page 41, details the cost of purchasing and operating alternative A for each year, for a period of 10 years. As the equipment has to be purchased before

Table 9. Life-Cycle Cost for Meal Assembly Line Replacement: Alternative A

		Life-Cycle Costs, $						
Year	Equipment Cost	Salaries, 10% Annual Increase	Supplies, 12% Annual Increase	Maintenance, 15% Annual Increase	Allocated Overhead, 15% Annual Increase	Total	Present Value of $1 Due in N Period, $	Discounted Present Value at 14%, $
0	95,000	0	0	0	0	95,000	0	95,000
1	0	8,500	200	1,500	2,000	12,200	0.877	10,699
2	0	9,350	224	1,725	2,300	13,599	0.769	10,458
3	0	10,285	251	1,984	2,645	15,165	0.675	10,236
4	0	11,313	281	2,282	3,042	16,918	0.592	10,015
5	0	12,444	315	2,624	3,498	18,881	0.519	9,799
6	0	13,688	353	3,018	4,023	21,082	0.456	9,613
7	0	15,057	395	3,471	4,626	23,549	0.400	9,420
8	0	16,563	442	3,992	5,320	26,317	0.351	9,237
9	0	18,219	495	4,591	6,118	29,423	0.308	9,062
10	0	20,041	554	5,280	7,036	32,911	0.270	8,886
					Total life-cycle cost	305,045		192,425

Capital Investment Analysis ■ 41

the meal assembly line can be operated, the $95,000 expenditure is not discounted and is carried out at full value. In the first year of operation, the total operating cost for salary, supply, maintenance, and allocated overhead costs amounted to $12,200. The present value of $1 due in one year is $0.877, as shown in table 10, below, under the 14 percent column. Thus, the present value of $12,200 for one year at 14 percent is $10,699. In the second year, it is estimated that the total operating cost for salary, supply, maintenance, and allocated overhead costs increased by 10 percent, 12 percent, 15 percent, and 15 percent, respectively. The total operating expenses for the second year amounted to $13,599 and was discounted to $10,458. This process is continued for the next eight years. The total life-cycle cost for alternative A is $305,045 and $192,425 when discounted at the present value rate of 14 percent. On the same basis, table 11, page 43, outlines the cost of purchasing and operating alternative B at $316,007 with a discounted present value of $168,053.

Now the food service administrator is in a position to evaluate the financial feasibility of these two alternatives. Table 12, page 44, which summarizes the life-cycle costs of alternatives A and B, demonstrates that alternative B is a more favorable capital expenditure.

Comparison of Alternatives

Discounted cash flow analysis can be used extensively to assist food service adminstrators in choosing from among various proposed capital expenditures. By facilitating the ranking of various capital expenditure projects on the basis of net present value, this approach enhances the selection process and the food service administrator is able to compare two or more alternatives on the same basis and select the most economical one. This approach ensures that scarce resources are equitably allocated and are efficiently utilized in the management of the project or program.

Objective Criteria

The reasons for increased need for objective criteria can be summarized as follows:

■ Increased advances in technology and decreased availability of funds enhance the sharp competition for resources in the health care field.

Table 10. Present Value of $1.00 Due in N Periods, Selected Values

Period, Years	Interest Rate			
	8%	14%	16%	20%
1	0.926	0.877	0.862	0.833
2	0.857	0.769	0.743	0.694
3	0.794	0.675	0.641	0.579
4	0.735	0.592	0.552	0.482
5	0.681	0.519	0.476	0.402
6	0.830	0.456	0.410	0.335
7	0.583	0.400	0.354	0.279
8	0.540	0.351	0.305	0.233
9	0.500	0.308	0.263	0.194
10	0.463	0.270	0.227	0.162
11	0.429	0.237	0.195	0.135
12	0.397	0.208	0.168	0.112
13	0.368	0.182	0.145	0.093
14	0.340	0.160	0.125	0.078
15	0.315	0.140	0.108	0.065

Table 11. Life-Cycle Cost for Meal Assembly Line Replacement: Alternative B

Life-Cycle Costs, $

Year	Equipment Cost	Salaries, 10% Annual Increase	Supplies, 12% Annual Increase	Maintenance, 15% Annual Increase	Allocated Overhead, 15% Annual Increase	Total	Present Value of $1 Due in N Period, $	Discounted Present Value at 14%, $
0	40,000	0	0	0	0	40,000	0	40,000
1	0	11,200	350	2,500	2,000	16,050	0.877	14,076
2	0	12,320	392	2,875	2,300	17,887	0.769	13,755
3	0	13,552	439	3,306	2,645	19,942	0.675	13,461
4	0	14,907	492	3,802	3,042	22,243	0.592	13,168
5	0	16,398	551	4,372	3,498	24,819	0.519	12,881
6	0	18,038	617	5,028	4,023	27,706	0.456	12,634
7	0	19,842	691	5,782	4,626	30,941	0.400	12,376
8	0	21,826	774	6,649	5,320	34,569	0.351	12,134
9	0	24,009	867	7,646	6,118	38,640	0.308	11,901
10	0	26,410	971	8,793	7,036	43,210	0.270	11,667
					Total life-cycle cost	316,007		168,053

Table 12. Summary of Life-Cycle Costs for Alternatives A and B

Alternative	Initial Equipment Cost, $	Initial Investment Savings, $	10-Year Life-Cycle Cost, $	Life-Cycle Savings, $
A	95,000		192,425	
B	40,000		168,053	
A − B		55,000		24,372

Note: Alternative B appears to be a more favorable capital expenditure because its life-cycle savings is $24,372 more than Alternative A.

■ Objective evaluations detail the impact of expenditures on future operations and cash outlays over an extended period of time.
■ The increasing role of government in monitoring and controlling health care costs requires health care institutions to contain costs and to be managed efficiently.
■ Objective financial evaluations are considered by most administrators to be prudent business practice.

Bibliography

Berman, Howard J., and Weeks, Lewis E. *The Financial Management of Hospitals.* 5th ed. Ann Arbor, MI: Health Administration Press, 1981.

Cleverley, William O. *Financial Management of Health Care Facilities.* Germantown, MD: Aspen Systems Corp., 1976.

Griffith, John R. *Quantitative Techniques for Hospital Planning and Control.* Lexington, MA: D. C. Heath & Company, 1972.

Herkimer Jr., Allen G. *Understanding Hospital Financial Management.* Germantown, MD: Aspen Systems Corp., 1978.

Keiser, James, and Kallio, Elmer. *Controlling and Analyzing Costs in Food Service Operations:* New York City: John Wiley & Sons, Inc., 1974.

Figure 9. Sample Form for Evaluation of Capital Equipment Requests

Capital Equipment Request

Department _____
Submitted by _____

Equipment _____

1. Intended use

   A. Give a general description of the intended use of the equipment.
   _____
   _____
   _____

   B. What departments or types of patients will benefit most by the use of this equipment? _____
   _____
   _____

   C. List possible alternatives to the requested equipment (purchase, lease, share). _____
   _____
   _____

   D. Will this equipment be viewed by the Health Planning Council as a change in service?
   Yes _____ No _____

   E. Priority: When is the equipment needed? _____   _____
                                                  Month   Year
   Is equipment: Urgent _____ Essential _____ Desirable _____

   Was equipment specified on your three-year capital equipment plan?   Yes _____ No _____

   Was the equipment included in the final approved budget for the fiscal year?
   _____
   _____

2. Financial justification
   A. Purchase—one time expenditures
      1. Cost of equipment $_____
      2. Cost of equipment accessories   _____
      3. Installation (in-house or outside vendor)   _____
      4. Remodeling (in-house or outside vendor)   _____
      5. Anticipated life of equipment   _____
      6. Estimated annual depreciation of purchase   _____
      Total $_____
   B. Effect on annual operations; increase (decrease) from current status
      1. Revenue (change in volume at average charge) $_____
      2. Salaries and fringes
         a. Number of FTE × average salary   _____
         b. Reclassification effect (if any)   _____
      3. Other operating expenses   _____
      4. Increase (decrease) in cost of other hospital departments   _____
      5. Annual maintenance (in-house or outside vendor)   _____
      6. Estimated annual depreciation of purchase (line 2A.6, above)   _____
      Total $_____
   C. Other Items
      1. Initial inventory—estimate $_____
      2. Salvage value of replaced equipment   _____
      3. Miscellaneous (specify) _____   _____

Evaluation of Cost-Allocation Methods

Chapter 4

One of the most compelling reasons for instituting a process to identify and apportion costs within the food service department is the complex nature of food service activity. It is a multiproduct service catering to two distinct and different clients: patients and nonpatients.

The patient component provides clinical nutrition services and a complete meal service, including nourishment and supplemental feeding programs. The nonpatient component encompasses the cafeteria, coffee shop, catering functions, and vending operations. It is experiencing an accelerated growth in revenue and in menu offerings and is attracting a wide variety of patrons who appreciate good-quality meal service at a competitive price. At present, the nonpatient food service of a number of health care institutions is actively competing with commercial restaurants in providing a high-quality menu and well-decorated and pleasant environment that are conducive to staff and employee enjoyment and relaxation. The staffing pattern for growth in nonpatient food service, then, must be significantly different from that in patient food service in such areas as preparation, delivery, merchandising, and presentation of the product.

Another factor influencing the need to determine and to allocate costs between patient and nonpatient food service is the larger allocation of resources required by the patient food service because of its unique delivery system and complexity of diets. Given the current emphasis on cost containment, the prospect of a change in hospital reimbursement methods to prospective payments for Medicare patients, and reliance on the competitive forces in the marketplace, it is important for the food service administrator to identify the precise cost of a unit of service and to manage the department with a defined cost pattern.

Finally, from a management perspective, it is important to differentiate the various nonpatient food service costs, such as the cafeteria, coffee shop, catering, and vending operations, to properly allocate resources to personnel, materials, and capital expenditure.

The *Determination and Allocation of Food Service Costs*[1] is an excellent reference book for a review of the basic concept of cost apportionment. There are four major methods of determining and allocating food service department costs. Familiarity with and the practice of these four approaches provide the food service administrator with an effective tool for managing the food service department. Each method has its own characteristics, which reflect its scope and accuracy and the level of sophistication of the data. These four methods are based on:

- Percent distribution of patient and nonpatient meals
- Direct allocation of costs, plus volume variable for centralized activities
- Labor costs of centralized activities, cafeteria, and patient meal service
- Meal equivalents

Although the above methods of cost allocation have been identified as vital to the integrity of the cost accounting, there is no assurance that following one of these methods will guarantee a successful operation without adhering to a well-defined management plan. However, identification of costs for the various activities does facilitate collection of relevant information that will enable the food service administrator to make better decisions.

Percentage Distribution of Patient and Nonpatient Meals

Determination of the percentage distribution of patient and nonpatient meals is a simple method for identifying and collecting costs. At the outset, it is essential to define a unit of service. Traditionally, the food service department has determined its unit of service to be one meal served to a patient or nonpatient. The number of meals served reflects the level of activity and the resources necessary to produce such a service.

The number of patient meals served is determined by counting all the meals served to an inpatient at regular mealtimes. The American Hospital Association's Hospital Administrative Services (HAS) suggests that a hospital with a 5-meal plan should report inpatient meals at 2.8 meals per patient day. Also, nourishments, tube feedings, and infant formulas should be excluded from these two calculations. It is further suggested that an accurate accounting method be instituted to capture the costs of nourishments. The cost for this service would then be divided by the patient days. Whereas the cost of prescribed nourishment, such as milk shakes, ice creams, juices, and sandwiches, usually is considered part of the patient meal cost, that of routine nourishment should be treated separately.

Determination of the percent distribution of patient and nonpatient meals is illustrated in the following example:

Type	Number of Meals	Percentage
Patient	37,325	49
Nonpatient	38,850	51
Total	76,175	100

The percentage of patient meals is determined by dividing patient meals (37,325) by the total department meals (76,175), resulting in 49 percent of the department resources being devoted to patient activity. To arrive at the nonpatient meal percentage, either subtract 49 percent from 100 percent or divide nonpatient meals (38,850) by the total department meals (76,175). Thus, the total unit of service and the percentage distribution of patient and nonpatient activities have been defined and identified.

Assignment of total department costs is made on the basis of individual patient and nonpatient percentages. The following example illustrates how the total department costs of $380,875 for food, labor, supply, and other are allocated on the basis of the percentage distribution of patient and nonpatient meals.

Expense	Total Department, 100%	Patient, 49%	Nonpatient, 51%
Food	$125,689	$ 61,588	$ 64,101
Labor	228,525	111,977	116,548
Supply	19,044	9,332	9,712
Other	7,617	3,732	3,885
Total	$380,875	$186,629	$194,246

Cost per meal is calculated by dividing the total department costs ($380,875) by the total department meals (76,175), resulting in $5.00 per meal. The same method of calculation is applied to determine the per meal costs of the other expense items. For example, food costs per meal are determined by dividing total department food costs ($125,689) by total department meals ($76,175) resulting in $1.65 per meal food cost.

Expense	Total Department	Patient	Nonpatient
Food	$1.65	$1.65	$1.65
Labor	3.00	3.00	3.00
Supply	.25	.25	.25
Other	.10	.10	.10
Total	$5.00	$5.00	$5.00

This is a simple way to divide food service department costs and arrive at a meal cost. The major weakness of this application is that the cost per meal is averaged between patient and nonpatient food service activities. It equalizes the operating costs of food, labor, supply, and other between the two major activities, rather than differentiating and assigning costs on the basis of the resources expended for each activity. Clearly the patient cost assignment for food was overstated, and the remaining costs for labor, supply, and other were understated. These disadvantages should be recognized by anyone using this method of apportioning costs.

Direct Allocation of Costs, plus Volume Variable

The second major approach to determining and allocating food service department costs is direct allocation of costs and application of the volume variable (unit of service) to apportion the operating costs of centralized activities. The food service department has a number of functions that result in both patient and nonpatient services, such as purchasing, receiving, storage, ingredient room (commissary), hot and cold food production, dishwashing, and sanitation. For the purpose of this calculation, these functions are classified as centralized food service activities. They are centrally organized for efficiency, cost savings, and quality control. The costs for these activities can be allocated on the basis of their percentage of either total department meals or total volume of centralized production.

Total Department Meals

A method to apportion the cost of centralized food service activities based on the percentage distribution of patient and nonpatient meals is as follows. First, the food service department record reflects the number of meals and the percentage distribution of patient and nonpatient meals.

Type	Meals	Percentage
Patient	37,325	49
Nonpatient	38,850	51
Total	76,175	100

The next step in this process is to review the operating expense accounts and ascertain the proper charges for food, labor, supply, and other miscellaneous costs. At the time of purchase the administrator should be able to identify the particular use of a product, that is, whether it will be used for patient or nonpatient functions. For example, patient service offers ice cream in 4-ounce containers, whereas nonpatient service purchases ice cream in 2½-gallon containers. The same approach is used for dietary supplies. For example, patient service uses place mats and two-ply napkins, whereas nonpatient service does not use place mats and uses only one-ply napkins.

Another method of identification between the expenses of two or more cost centers is the use of requisitions to order products and supplies from a central storeroom or a commissary. Also, labor costs can be easily captured for those employees who are primarily working in patient meal service or in the cafeteria. These types of costs can be identified and fairly assigned to the particular cost center. The following example provides information on total department costs, assigned operating costs to patient and nonpatient services, and centralized activities costs.

Expense	Total Department	Patient Assigned	Nonpatient Assigned	Centralized Activities
Food	$125,689	$ 20,000	$ 35,000	$ 70,689
Labor	228,525	115,000	65,000	48,525
Supply	19,044	9,500	6,500	3,044
Other	7,617	3,000	2,500	2,117
Total	$380,875	$147,500	$109,000	$124,375

Next, the costs of the centralized food service activities should be apportioned on the basis of the percentage distribution of patient and nonpatient meals. This calculation is made to reflect the level of activity and expenditure.

Expense	Centralized Activities, 100%	Patient, 49%	Nonpatient, 51%
Food	$ 70,689	$34,638	$36,051
Labor	48,525	23,777	24,748
Supply	3,044	1,492	1,552
Other	2,117	1,037	1,080
Total	$124,375	$60,944	$63,431

The total food service department cost allocation by percentage distribution of patient and nonpatient meals is summarized in table 13, below.

The cost per meal for the food service department is:

Expense	Total Department, 100%	Patient, 49%	Nonpatient, 51%
Food	$1.65	$1.46	$1.83
Labor	3.00	3.72	2.31
Supply	.25	.29	.21
Other	.10	.11	.09
Total	$5.00	$5.58	$4.44

Table 13. Cost Allocation Based on Centralized Food Service Activities as Determined by Meals

		Patient, $			Nonpatient, $		
Expense	Total Department, $	Assigned	Meals, 49%	Total	Assigned	Meals, 51%	Total
Food	125,689	20,000	34,638	54,638	35,000	36,051	71,051
Labor	228,525	115,000	23,777	138,777	65,000	24,748	89,748
Supply	19,044	9,500	1,492	10,992	6,500	1,552	8,052
Other	7,617	3,000	1,037	4,037	2,500	1,080	3,580
Total	380,875	147,500	60,944	208,444	109,000	63,431	172,431

Although the average cost per meal for the total department is $5, there are significant differences in food, labor, supply, and other expenses between the patient and nonpatient activities. The patient activities show a lower food cost than the nonpatient activities. This can be attributed to the HAS definition of an equivalent cafeteria meal compared with a patient meal that may not be complete because of restricted diet or lack of appetite. To ensure proper preparation of patient foods, handling, delivery, and nutritional assessment activities, labor costs are usually higher, reflecting the level of care. The supply and other costs also are higher for patients because of the aforementioned reasons. In summary, the operating costs for nonpatient activities are sometimes considered to be lower because of the nature and type of menu offered and the utilization of the self-service system.

Centralized Production Volume

Another way to allocate costs of the centralized food service activities is on the basis of percentage distribution of patient and nonpatient production volume, in which the food service department documents the number of food portions prepared in hot and cold food production for a specified period of time.

Type	Number of Portions	Percentage
Patient	37,611	45
Nonpatient	45,969	55
Total	83,580	100

It is noteworthy to acknowledge the different percentages that result from the two methods.

Type	Percentage Distribution Meals	Portions
Patient	49	45
Nonpatient	51	55
Total	100	100

The variance between the meals and portions is 4 percent. Patient service is 4 percent higher for meals than for portions. The variance between these two concepts is attributed to the fact that HAS has specifically defined the contents of an equivalent cafeteria meal, whereas patients have the option to select their meals from a menu or are restricted to a limited number of portions because of their particular diet. Given this variance in the method of apportionment, the food service administrator has to quantify these differences and relate them to the level of effort required to produce these menu items. Basically, this difference should be resolved in a fair manner between the two activities.

Costs of the centralized food service activities, allocated on the basis of percentage distribution of patient and nonpatient production volume, or portions, are:

Expense	Centralized Activities, 100%	Patient, 45%	Nonpatient, 55%
Food	$ 70,689	$31,810	$38,879
Labor	48,525	21,836	26,689
Supply	3,044	1,370	1,674
Other	2,117	953	1,164
Total	$124,375	$55,969	$68,406

The total food service department cost allocation by percentage distribution of patient and nonpatient portions is shown in table 14, below.

The cost per meal for the food service department is obtained as follows:

Expense	Total Department, 100%	Patient, 45%	Nonpatient, 55%
Food	$1.65	$1.39	$1.90
Labor	3.00	3.67	2.36
Supply	.25	.29	.21
Other	.10	.11	.09
Total	$5.00	$5.46	$4.56

Meals vs. Portions

The following illustrates the differences in cost per meal between the two approaches:

		Meals		Portions	
Expense	Total Department, 100%	Patient, 49%	Nonpatient, 51%	Patient, 45%	Nonpatient, 55%
Food	$1.65	$1.46	$1.83	$1.39	$1.90
Labor	3.00	3.72	2.31	3.67	2.36
Supply	.25	.29	.21	.29	.21
Other	.10	.11	.09	.11	.09
Total	$5.00	$5.58	$4.44	$5.46	$4.56

It is evident that the overall variance in meal costs between the two methods of allocation is only 2 percent, or 12 cents. Under the distribution of portions method, the nonpatient activity increased by 7 cents for food cost and 5 cents for labor per meal. The supply and other expenses remained constant for the two methods. In summary, the calculations suggest that the use of percentage distribution of portions, as produced by the centralized food service activity, is a more accurate indicator of resource allocation.

Labor Costs

A modern food service facility in a 555-bed teaching hospital was used in a study conducted (1) to determine the labor cost for a centralized food service activity, including such functions as purchasing, stores, forecasting, sanitation, and hot and cold food preparation, and (2) to assign a labor cost for each food portion produced.[2] Table 15, page 53, shows the components of the centralized production function and the labor minutes required for a typical day.

Column A, Menu Item, lists the types of items required to prepare the major ingredients of the menu.

Column B reflects the total portions that must be prepared for each menu item, for example, 650 portions of breakfast cookery.

Table 14. Cost Allocation Based on Centralized Food Service Activities as Determined by Portions

		Patient, $			Nonpatient, $		
Expense	Total Department, $	Assigned	Volume, 45%	Total	Assigned	Volume, 55%	Total
Food	125,689	20,000	31,810	51,810	35,000	38,879	73,879
Labor	228,525	115,000	21,836	136,836	65,000	26,689	91,689
Supply	19,044	9,500	1,370	10,870	6,500	1,674	8,174
Other	7,617	3,000	953	3,953	2,500	1,164	3,664
Total	380,875	147,500	55,969	203,469	109,000	68,406	177,406

Table 15. Labor Costs of Centralized Food Production

A Menu Item	B Total Portions	C Cook Labor, Minutes	D Work Labor, Minutes	E Labor Effort per Portion, RVU	F Total Effort, RVU (B × E)	G Labor Minutes Assigned by RVU	H Total Labor Minutes (C+D+G)	I Labor Minutes per Portion (H ÷ B)
Breakfast cookery	650	191		1.00	650	635	826	1.27
Soup	420	54		.25	105	103	157	.37
Entree	1,960	938		2.00	3,920	3,831	4,769	2.43
Gravy	760	48		.10	76	74	122	.16
Starch	740	59		.25	185	181	240	.32
Vegetable	890	88		.25	223	218	306	.34
Salad	1,776		480	.25	444	434	914	.51
Sandwich	612		720	.25	153	150	870	1.42
Dessert	550	62		.25	138	134	196	.36
Total	8,358	1,440	1,200	4.60	5,894	5,760	8,400	

Column C indicates the actual minutes it took to produce a menu item. For example, 191 minutes was devoted to the preparation of 650 portions of breakfast cookery.

Column D shows the number of minutes the food service employees were assigned to produce a specific menu item. For example, 480 minutes of food service worker time was spent to prepare 1,776 salads.

Column E shows the level of effort required to prepare a specific menu item and compares it with other efforts needed to prepare different menu items. For example, it took 1.00 relative value unit (RVU) to produce a portion of breakfast cookery compared to 2.00 RVUs to prepare one portion of an entree.

Column F reflects the total effort required to prepare a specific product for that day. For example, 650 portions of breakfast cookery (column B) multiplied by 1.00 RVU labor effort (column E) is 650 RVUs of total effort (column F).

The total minutes of 5,760 in column G represents food service workers assigned to multiple functions that cannot be ascertained easily. Their time is allocated to a menu item on the basis of total effort, as indicated in column F, in the amount of 5,894. To properly assign labor minutes to the specific menu items, a general ratio has to be determined for the total effort (5,894 RVUs, column F), total minutes of unassigned labor (5,760 minutes, column G), and the total effort for a specific menu item (for example, breakfast cookery in column F). The following calculation is then made: The total effort in column F for breakfast cookery, 650, is multiplied by 5,760 labor minutes, column G, and then divided by 5,894, total effort in column F, resulting in 635, as shown in column G.

Column H is the total amount of labor minutes, as shown in columns C, D, and G. For example, it took 826 labor minutes to prepare 650 portions of breakfast cookery.

Column I shows the calculated labor minutes for each menu item. For example, it took 1.27 minutes to produce one portion of breakfast cookery. The labor minute per portion as expressed in column I is important information that is required to allocate labor cost to patient and nonpatient food service activities.

But before labor costs can be allocated to either patient or nonpatient food service activities, the appropriate labor cost must be ascertained for each menu item sold in the cafeteria. Table 16, page 55, highlights the cafeteria menu items that are available on a typical day and the labor minutes required for the service and sale of these items. The same guidelines were followed in calculating labor minutes and RVUs. The conversion of the labor minutes into RVUs for a specific menu item was accomplished by multiplying the total portions for the specific item (column D) by the total labor minutes (column E) and dividing the result by total effort RVUs (column D). For example, the labor minutes assigned to the breakfast cookery as RVUs are calculated as follows:

$$\frac{275 \text{ RVUs} \times 8{,}579 \text{ Total labor minutes}}{4{,}407 \text{ Total RVUs}} = 535 \text{ Labor minutes}$$

This calculation is performed on all the cafeteria menu items in order to obtain an individual value for each item offered for sale (column E).

Finally, column F reflects the cafeteria labor minutes required to sell a portion of food from the menu. The food service administrator can analyze and compare the labor cost per menu item against both the daily sales and the monthly financial statement.

The administrator will be interested in ascertaining the total cafeteria labor cost for each menu item, to facilitate the cafeteria pricing function. Table 17, page 55, shows the following costs and how they are derived:

- Cafeteria labor minutes per menu item (column B)
- Centralized food production labor minutes per menu item (column C)
- Total cafeteria labor minutes per menu item (column D)
- Total labor cost per menu item offered for sale in the cafeteria (column E)

Table 16. Labor Costs of Cafeteria

A Menu Item	B Total Portion	C Labor Effort, RVU	D Total Effort, RVU (B×C)	E Labor Minutes Assigned by RVU	F Labor Minute per Portion (E÷B)
Breakfast cookery	275	1.00	275	535	1.945
Soup	220	.25	55	107	.486
Entree	1,245	2.00	2,490	4,848	3.894
Gravy	480	.10	48	93	.194
Starch	350	.25	88	171	.489
Vegetable	350	.25	88	171	.489
Salad	875	.25	219	426	.487
Sandwich	401	.25	100	195	.486
Dessert	408	.25	102	199	.488
Grilled items	685	1.00	685	1,334	1.95
Beverages	3,095	.05	155	302	.10
Ice cream	326	.15	49	95	.29
Cookies	275	.05	14	27	.10
Sweet roll	325	.05	16	31	.10
Fresh fruit	175	.05	9	18	.10
Miscellaneous	285	.05	14	27	.10
Total	9,770	6.00	4,407	8,579	

Table 17. Total Labor Costs of Cafeteria

A Menu Item	B Labor Minutes per Portion	C Production Labor Minutes per Portion	D Total Labor Minutes per Portion (B+C)	E Labor at $.1205 per Minute (D×.1205), $
Breakfast cookery	1.945	1.27	3.215	0.39
Soup	.486	.37	0.856	0.103
Entree	3.894	2.43	6.324	0.76
Gravy	.194	.16	0.354	0.043
Starch	.489	.32	0.809	0.10
Vegetable	.489	.34	0.829	0.10
Salad	.487	.51	0.997	0.12
Sandwich	.486	1.42	1.906	0.23
Dessert	.488	.36	0.848	0.102
Grilled items	1.95		1.95	0.234
Beverages	.10		.10	0.012
Ice cream	.29		.29	0.035
Cookies	.10		.10	0.012
Sweet roll	.10		.10	0.012
Fresh fruit	.10		.10	0.012
Miscellaneous	.10		.10	0.012

Patient meal service labor costs also can be studied on the basis of the guidelines provided in the previous paragraph. Table 18, below, shows the menu items, the number of portions, the RVUs, and the labor minutes assigned to each portion of the patient menu.

The total patient meal-service labor cost is summarized in table 19, page 57. A dollar value is assigned to each portion of food, and the amount of total labor minutes per portion of food is identified. This information is vital to the food service administrator's decision-making process because it pinpoints the estimated cost of labor for a particular service, such as patient meal, nourishment, and floor stocking.

The food service administrator is now able to use the labor cost for each food item produced or handled by the food service employees, together with food cost data, to make informed decisions without lowering the quality of care and service.

Meal Equivalents

The meal equivalent approach for allocating food service costs is fairly simple. The distribution of costs is determined by using a meal equivalent value and operating statement expense indicators or other desired percentages. For example, the average selling price of an equivalent meal in the cafeteria is $2.25, and the desired operating percentages are 51 percent for food cost, 42 percent for labor cost, and 6 percent for other costs. One percentage point is reserved for a net income over expenses. In an effort to calculate the values for food, labor, and other costs, the assumption is made that the average selling price of $2.25 equals 100 percent; then the expense percentages for food, labor, and other costs are calculated. Table 20, page 57, shows individual costs for each meal component of food, labor, and other.

To allocate cafeteria resources to the various operating expense accounts, the individual cost for each meal equivalent is multiplied by the total meal equivalent for the period in question, as shown in Table 21, page 58.

To obtain an equivalent meal count in a nonpatient food service activity (cafeteria), total sales should be divided by the average selling price of a full meal

Table 18. Labor Costs of Patient Meal Service

A Menu Item	B Total Portions	C Labor Effort, RVU	D Total Effort, RVU (B×C)	E Labor Minutes Assigned, by RVU	F Labor Minute per Portion (E÷B)
Breakfast cookery	375	.75	281	2,630	7.013
Soup	200	.25	50	468	2.340
Entree	715	.85	608	5,690	7.958
Gravy	280	.10	28	262	.936
Starch	390	.25	97	908	2.338
Vegetable	540	.25	135	1,263	2.339
Salad	901	.25	225	2,106	2.337
Sandwich	211	.15	32	299	1.417
Dessert	142	.25	35	328	2.310
Beverage	1,275	.05	64	599	.470
Ice cream	350	.10	35	328	.937
Juice	450	.05	22	206	.458
Cookies	325	.05	16	150	.461
Sweet roll	225	.05	11	103	.458
Fresh fruit	195	.05	10	94	.482
Dinner roll	750	.05	37	346	.461
Total	7,324	3.50	1,686	15,780	

Table 19. Total Labor Costs of Patient Meal Service

A Menu Item	B Labor Minutes per Portion	C Production Labor Minutes per Portion	D Total Labor Minutes per Portion (B+C)	E Labor at $.1205 per Minute (D×.1205), $
Breakfast cookery	7.013	1.27	8.283	0.998
Soup	2.340	.37	2.710	0.326
Entree	7.958	2.43	10.388	1.252
Gravy	.936	.16	1.096	0.132
Starch	2.328	.32	2.648	0.319
Vegetable	2.339	.34	2.679	0.323
Salad	2.337	.51	2.847	0.343
Sandwich	1.417	1.42	2.837	0.342
Dessert	2.310	.36	2.670	0.322
Beverage	.470		.470	0.057
Ice cream	.937		.937	0.113
Juice	.458		.458	0.055
Cookies	.461		.461	0.055
Sweet roll	.458		.458	0.055
Fresh fruit	.482		.482	0.058
Dinner roll	.461		.461	0.055

Table 20. Cost Allocation for Cafeteria Based on Meal Equivalent and Operating Expense

Meal Component	Selling Price	Food Cost, $	Labor Cost, $	Other Cost, $	Total Costs, $
Meat	1.10	0.561	0.462	0.066	1.089
Potato	.20	.102	.084	.012	.198
Vegetable	.20	.102	.084	.012	.198
Salad	.40	.204	.168	.024	.396
Beverage	.10	.051	.042	.006	.099
Dessert	.25	.127	.105	.015	.247
Total	2.25	1.147	0.945	0.135	2.227
Operating statement or desired percentages	100%	51%	42%	6%	99%

Table 21. Cost Allocation of Cafeteria Resources

A Expense	B Cost per Meal Equivalent, $	C Meal Equivalent	D Total Cost (B×C), $
Food	1.147	38,850	44,561
Labor	0.945	38,850	36,713
Other	0.135	38,850	5,245
Total costs	2.227	38,850	86,519

served at noon. HAS defines the components of an equivalent full meal as meat, potato, vegetable, salad, beverage, and dessert. When there is a selection of entrees, starches, vegetables, salads, desserts, and so forth that are available at different prices, an average price should be used in calculating the selling price of a full meal. Although HAS does not specify a method to calculate a catering meal equivalent, it is suggested that, to obtain an equivalent meal count for catered events, total catered sales should be divided by the average selling price of a full meal served in the cafeteria at noon. This technique slightly inflates the number of equivalent meals, but it is justified because catered events do require greater resources for food, labor, and supply costs than are required for cafeteria meals.

The meal equivalent approach is rarely used alone. This approach is used as a guideline and for verification along with other resource allocation methods.

Notes

[1] American Hospital Association. *Determination of the Food Service Costs.* Chicago: AHA, 1976.

[2] Kaud, F. A. A Study of Labor Costs of Centralized Food Service Activities, The Cafeteria and Patient Meal Service. Unpublished study, June 1981.

Management of the Clinical Dietetics Staff

Chapter 5

Over the past 10 years, the image of the dietitian's role has changed from a limited one to that of a full-fledged member of the health care team. Advances in technology, higher educational requirements, and the general swing toward preventive medicine have all contributed to this expanded role.

The political environment also affects the dietitian's status. Because of the changing regulatory environment, it is clear that the food service administrator in conjunction with the clinical dietary staff must develop strategies to ensure that high-quality nutritional care is provided at a competitive rate in an era of limited resources. Alex McMahon, president, American Hospital Association, succinctly summarized the effect of President Reagan's goal of balancing the federal budget: "(Health care) costs will be reduced whether through regulation or competition."[1]

Function of the Hospital Clinical Dietitian

To delineate adequately the function of the clinical dietitian in the hospital setting, the food service administrator may wish to refer to the Joint Commission on Accreditation of Hospitals (JCAH) requirements for dietary services. The primary principle as defined by the JCAH is to meet adequately the nutritional needs of patients, for which purpose the *Accreditation Manual for Hospitals*[2] recommends that certain standards be met. The following is a summary of the essential functions of the clinical dietitian[3]:

1. Nutrition assessment and development of a care plan

- Analyze patient's ability to consume food (patient visitation at meal time)
- Review patient's medical record
- Review patient's current medical status through patient visitation, chart review, interdisciplinary team conferences, consultation with other staff, and so forth
- Prepare nutritional care plan and analyze actual intake (calorie counts and so forth)

2. Patient education

- Instruct patients regarding therapeutic diets and/or normal nutrition
- Refer patients to local health agency or primary care physician, outlining the nutritional care provided

3. Documentation in the medical record

- Record nutrition assessment and nutritional care plan
- Describe patient education conducted, evaluate level of patient's understanding, list further education recommended, and document referral to other practitioners/sources

4. Menus evaluated for nutritional adequacy and/or adherence to diet order

- Review nontherapeutic diets for nutritional adequacy (review menus)
- Evaluate therapeutic diets for nutritional adequacy and adherence to diet order (write menus)

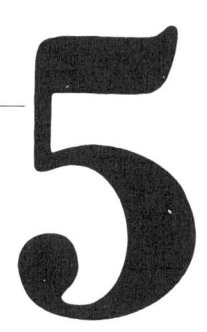

5. Job-related activities

- Continue professional development (continuing education)
- Educate dietetic interns, technicians, food service workers, and diet clerks
- Conduct in-service education of other health care team members
- Review diet manual/handbook
- Participate in quality assurance program
- Prepare reports
- Evaluate the meal service
- Review policy and procedures

In an effort to facilitate the fulfillment of these responsibilities, the hospital clinical dietitian and the dietetic technician (a graduate of a two-year nutrition program) are evaluated according to objectives and tasks delineated for dietitians and dietetic technicians. Sample position descriptions are shown in figures 10 and 11, following this chapter. These descriptions were developed on the basis of department goals and actual job performance.

Measuring Performance

The preceding paragraphs emphasize the need to properly identify the role of the hospital clinical dietitian and to differentiate it from actual responsibilities for food preparation, assembly, and meal service.

It is suggested that the number of meals served per paid hour does not adequately measure hospital food service department productivity because it measures the preparation and service of a patient meal, but does not take into account the professional services of the clinical dietary staff. Therefore, it is recommended that the hospital food service department measurement be expanded to include two important elements: clinical dietetics paid hours per patient day and clinical dietetics salary and benefit costs per patient day.

The equation for the clinical paid hours should include only professional staff services involved in delivering dietetic and nutritional care to patients. The staff may include dietitians, dietetic technicians (graduates of two-year dietetic training), and dietetic interns, if they provide patients with dietetic services. The functions of menu distribution and diet changes are considered to be part of serving a meal.

The next step in this evaluative process is to select a suitable performance measure to properly account for the hospital clinical dietitian's activities. Three general approaches to assess the level of nutritional care and define the cost of the clinical dietitian's service are mentioned below. The first two approaches are described briefly to acquaint the student of hospital food service administration with performance measure systems. The third approach—the time-task allocation method—is recommended because it is both easy and inexpensive and is, therefore, described in depth to document its proper use, cost, and benefits.

1. A plan proposed by Walters and others[4] make it possible to specify the scope of nutritional services for each hospitalized patient depending on his or her individual need, the type of personnel designated to perform the service, the time required to perform it, and the equation to convert the service into cost.

2. A system of relative value units (RVUs) is crucial to the establishment of a uniform accountability system. The RVU is used to compare the time required to perform specified, uniformly defined tasks encompassed by the clinical dietitian's functions, and enables the quantification, reporting, and comparison of performance outputs. It permits the identification of both specific, task-related costs as well as the total cost for the clinical dietetics department. Figure 12, following this chapter, presents a sample approach to RVUs in the clinical dietary service; as developed by Kaud and Becker, this method calculates RVUs on the basis of the estimated RVUs assigned to some basic dietary functions.[5] It is suggested that

food service administrators conduct their own work sampling studies to determine acceptable RVUs for the tasks performed by the clinical dietary service. The level of performance and, therefore, the assigned RVUs reflect the scope of nutrition assessment required in basic, intermediate, and complex levels of service.

To develop, implement, maintain, and monitor an RVU system for a specific clinical dietetics department, a complex system of accounting and record keeping is required. But, with the advent of minicomputers and other systems, it is now feasible and cost-effective to do so.

3. The time-task allocation method analyzes the major activities of a job and assigns a unit of time to each task. The assignment of time is based on a study of employees performing the specific function or through the accumulation of performance data from incumbent employees. The latter method uses employee performance reports to document the various activities. This approach requires three important elements:

- A detailed job description
- Specific and measurable objectives
- The clinical dietetics weekly status report (shown in figure 13, following this chapter)

The process operates as follows. A clinical dietitian, a technician, and a dietetic intern are assigned to a specific patient care unit. For example, in a university-based teaching hospital the staffing pattern of dietitians and dietetic technicians may be delineated as follows[6]:

- Trauma and burn units with average census of 12.7—0.5 FTE dietitian
- Oncology units with average census of 43.9—1.0 FTE dietitian
- Cardiovascular, cardiovascular surgery, surgery ICU, and anorexia nervosa units with average census of 41.3—1.0 FTE dietitian, 0.67 FTE technician
- Pediatrics with average census of 41.7—1.0 FTE dietitian, 1.0 FTE technician
- Surgery units with average census of 76.1—1.0 FTE dietitian, 0.33 FTE technician
- Renal, dialysis, and medical ICU units with average census of 43.4—1.0 FTE dietitian
- Rehabilitation and orthopedic surgery units with average census of 45.9—1.0 FTE dietitian
- General medicine, endocrinology, and gynecology with average census of 65.8—1.0 FTE dietitian, 1.0 FTE technician
- Special surgery and psychiatric units with average census of 49.0—1.0 FTE dietitian

In addition, dietetic interns rotate through each of these services according to a predetermined schedule.

A diet status report (shown in figure 14, following this chapter) is generated daily for each patient care unit. It contains the following basic information: room number, patient's name, diet order for dinner, breakfast, and lunch, and remarks. In some institutions, this report is generated by a computer or other mechanical device; it is prepared in quadruplicate and delivered to each patient care unit. The nursing unit clerk updates the pertinent patient information and, at two specific times of the day, dispatches the appropriate diet status report to the dietetics department. In addition to diet changes, the report contains information on admissions, transfers, and discharge. One copy of this diet status report is used by nursing personnel to verify diets at meal time, and the other copy is used by the clinical dietetics staff to keep track of patients' diets, patients visited, charting, and so forth. In addition, the clinical dietary staff receives a copy of the patient census sheet for each unit. This report includes each patient's name, age, sex, staff physician, service, and length of stay.

As each dietitian, technician, and dietetic intern makes a daily record of his or her activities in the weekly status report (figure 13, following this chapter), indicating the amount of time that was devoted to each segment of his or her assigned responsibilities, the director of clinical dietetics is able to examine the performance of the clinical dietetics staff members and also to assign the necessary resources to meet institutional and dietary department objectives.[7] The director of clinical dietetics is able to review each dietitian's, technician's, and dietetic intern's performance on a weekly basis and to compare it to preestablished objectives. For example, the distinction is made on the form between diets written and diets checked to ensure that therapeutic and general diet menus are monitored for nutritional adequacy. The major duties recorded on this form are compiled weekly to provide summary information. The clinical dietetics director can utilize this summary to evaluate the performance of the department, as well as for budget preparation. Also, the percentage of patients visited can be readily calculated from the number-of-patient-days data. To ensure the accuracy of the compiled data, it is important that the director of clinical dietetics and the clinical dietary staff members clearly define what will be included in each section of the weekly status report.

Using Time-Task Allocation for Management

The clinical dietetics weekly status report provides clear accountability for allocating resources and enables the department director to effectively review each staff member's performance according to preestablished objectives.

These objectives should be reviewed yearly as part of a staff member's annual performance review. If job duties change during the year, the relevant objectives must also be revised. How each staff member meets assigned, specific objectives then can be discussed with that individual on a quarterly basis. For example, the weekly objectives set for a clinical dietitian who works with a dietetic technician on the surgery units would be:

Nutrition assessment	17.5 hours	(47%)
Menus	1.0	(3)
Charting in medical records	5.0	(13)
Patient education	9.0	(24)
Other job-related activities	5.0	(13)
Total hours worked	37.5 hours	(100%)
Scheduled breaks	2.5	
Total paid hours	40.0 hours	

The summary of the clinical dietary department report (as shown in figure 15, following this chapter) enables the director to review the total activity of the department and to calculate the cost of the clinical dietetics staff. The report shows that the staff, which includes dietitians, dietetic technicians, and dietetic interns, spent 83 percent of their time providing direct patient care: nutrition assessment (32 percent), reviewing menus for nutritional adequacy (30 percent), charting in the medical record (11 percent), and patient education (10 percent). The remaining 16 percent of the clinical dietary staff time was spent on other job-related activities, such as professional development, dietetic intern teaching, meetings, record keeping, projects, and other similar tasks. This percentage should be examined from time to time to ensure adequate distribution of resources. A similar report, a sample of which appears in figure 16, following this chapter, illustrates the major responsibilities of the outpatient dietitian and how resources may be expended in this service area.

It is important that the food service administrator establish a method to determine the cost of this service to the institution and to the patient. For example, the cost of salary plus fringe benefits (approximately 26 percent of salary) can be computed as follows:

8.50 dietitians at $1,910 per month	$16,235
3.00 dietetic technicians at $1,570 per month	4,710
3.80 dietetic interns at $532 per month	2,021
15.30 total salary expense per month	$22,966

The average salary plus fringe benefits per hour is: $22,966 ÷ 15.3 FTEs ÷ 173.33 hours paid per month = $8.66.

The food service administrator may wish to assign a cost factor for the five major responsibilities of the clinical dietary department listed in figure 15. The weekly costs may be shown as follows:

Nutrition assessment	185.4 hours	×	$8.66	=	$1,605
Menu review	174.1	×	$8.66	=	1,508
Charting	63.5	×	$8.66	=	550
Patient education	58.2	×	$8.66	=	504
Other activities	95.0	×	$8.66	=	823
Breaks, vacation, sick leave	35.8	×	$8.66	=	310
Total paid hours	612.0 hours				$5,300

Another approach to calculating the cost of the clinical dietetic department uses the following factors:

■ Productive work minutes per patient day
■ Paid minutes per patient day
■ Salary and benefit costs per patient day

Assuming that patient days were 3,178 for the period in question, that is, one week, productive work minutes per patient day = 612 paid hours − 35.8 hours for breaks, vacation, and sick leave × 60 minutes ÷ 3,178 patient days = 10.88 productive work minutes per patient day. Salary and benefits costs per patient day = $5,300 ÷ 3,178 = $1.67 per patient day.

In conjunction with any productivity evaluation, the measure of the quality of the task performed is equally important, and various methods can be used for this. Chart audits performed either concurrently or retrospectively will provide information as to the quality of the documentation and also will provide an indication of the quality of care provided. Various quality assurance programs that are intended to ascertain quality of documentation have been reported in the literature.[8-10]

In addition, the director of clinical dietetics should routinely review all staff members' written menus and patient care plans, make patient meal rounds with them, observe various patient education sessions, and so forth. This direct observation, utilizing preestablished criteria, will help ensure high-quality care. Of course, the patients' understanding and adherence to their diets after discharge is the ultimate review of the quality of patient education. With all forms of quality review, it is imperative to use preestablished criteria and to review the results objectively with all members of the clinical dietetics staff; corrective action should be outlined in advance and taken when it is warranted.

Another method of evaluating the quality of staff performance is to review patient questionnaires. A typical postdischarge patient questionnaire includes two questions related to the quality of nutritional care received by the patient: "Were your questions on nutrition answered in a satisfactory manner?" and "If you were on a modified diet, was it satisfactorily explained to you?" The answers to these two questions are important indicators of a patient's perception of the care received.

Finally, an in-house food service department questionnaire may be distributed to all patients on a scheduled basis. This schedule is developed on the basis of random numbers, which facilitates sending the questionnaires on different days of the menu cycle and at different meals. The questionnaire asks the patient: "Did a dietitian or a technician visit you?" and "If you are on a modified diet, has it been explained to you by a dietitian or a dietetic technician?" The answers to these questions will also help identify a patient's perception of nutritional care received.

Using Time-Task Allocation for Budget Preparation

In addition to the benefit of establishing a specific objective for the individual dietitian, technician, and intern, the information generated from the weekly status report of the clinical dietetics department can be summarized and maintained on a monthly and yearly basis. This type of information becomes essential for budget preparation, at which time personnel activities and standards of clinical dietary care are used, particularly in projecting an increase or decrease in patient days. Figure 17, following this chapter, illustrates how the productivity and the standard of clinical dietetics care can operate effectively in determining the number of personnel required and at what level of care the clinical dietetics department is expected to function efficiently.

On the basis of information presented in this manner, the director of dietary services and the hospital administrator can effectively review what is being accomplished. In the example presented in figure 17A, this institution budgeted increased resources from 1980-81 to 1981-82, as reflected in columns 2 and 6, line H, which show an increase in number of FTEs from 12.28 to 13.94. This allowed for an increase in services, as follows:

- The percentage of patients visited increased from 88 percent in 1980-81 to 98 percent in 1981-82, as shown in columns 4 and 8, line A1.
- The percentage of medical records that contained a nutrition note increased from 28 percent in 1980-81 to 40 percent in 1981-82, as shown in columns 5 and 9, line C.
- The number of patients instructed weekly also increased from 54.7 hours in 1980-81 to 57.4 hours in 1981-82, as shown in columns 3 and 7, line B1.

Thus, it was possible to document what the increased budget expenditure had provided.

Also, the budget preparation process that utilizes the time-task allocation methodology allows the director of clinical dietetics to develop measurable productivity standards. For example, charting in medical records was forecast to increase from 68 percent of total admissions (Current Staffing) to 95 percent (Improved Service) in 1982-83, as shown in figure 17B, columns 5 and 9, line C. Meeting this goal will require that the director of clinical dietetics develop specific implementation plans, which could include an in-service education program, reevaluation of appropriate nutrition note content, development of a weekly monitoring system, and so forth.

The time-task allocation approach can be used to illustrate what effects a staff reduction would have on patient care. For example, if the number of FTEs were to be decreased by two, the director of clinical dietetics could provide the administrator with data indicating how the services provided to patients would be affected. Although the clinical dietetic staff would continue to function, it would be at the expense of lowering the compliance with various performance criteria. The director of clinical dietetics, the food service administrator, and the hospital administrator cannot claim such a change increases efficiency or contains costs without also accounting for the decrease in the amount of patient care being provided.

There is also the option of increasing the level of these performance criteria so as to attain a higher level of compliance with JCAH standards and the goals of the institution.

■ Nutrition assessment: increase the percentage of total patients visited to 98 percent (figure 17A, column 8, line A1)
■ Charting: increase the activity to 95 percent of admissions charted (figure 17B, column 9, line C)
■ Menu review for nutritional adequacy: attain a 54 percent review of all menus (figure 17B, column 8, line D2)
■ Other activities: maintain 95.0 hours for professional development and other job-related activities (figure 17B, column 7, line E)

Figure 17A and B, columns 6 and 7, shows the assignment of activities at an increased level of performance and productivity. It is clear, then, that the maintenance of such nutritional standards of care will require additional staff.

The next step in the budget preparation process would be to define the composition of the 3.52-FTE increase from 1980-81 to 1982-83: how many dietitians, dietetic technicians, and dietetic interns should be recruited? The answer to this question depends on a projection of the impact of recommended standards on each dietitian and technician, taking into account the goals of the institution or department, the training of potential employees, the unit preferences of current staff members, the length of patient stay, and the occupancy rate of each unit.

Cost Effectiveness of the Management Information System

There is a definite cost associated with maintaining clinical dietetics performance data for use in management decision making. The cost in terms of dollars and cents could vary significantly according to the type and accuracy of data collection methods and systems. This process involves a change in the behavior and attitude of the clinical dietetic staff, because it requires them to account for their performance in a consistent and measurable fashion. The collection of data necessary for management information purposes is time consuming and requires a concerted effort and considerable record keeping.

On the positive side of the equation, the process is an effective, manageable, and simple approach to providing the documentation necessary for the following activities:

■ **Performance evaluation.** The process facilitates the accomplishment of a clinical dietetics staff's daily objectives and provides a record of performance to be used in annual performance evaluation and in measuring performance against preestablished task objectives.
■ **Department evaluation.** This information assists the directors of clinical dietetic staff and the food service administrators in evaluating staffing patterns for current levels of activity, for new programs, or for changes in the levels of activity. Clearly, the clinical dietetics performance data can be conveniently and effectively utilized in the justification of the annual budget report and its various essential components.
■ **Planning.** The clinical dietetics management information system becomes a valuable tool when the health care institution is planning to build a new facility or expand or renovate an existing one. Also, this information may be of value to local health planning agencies when the health care institution requests approval for new construction or programs.
■ **Third-party reimbursement.** The availability of this clinical dietetics management information data enhances and documents the basis for third-party reimbursement of patient nutritional care.

On balance, the advantages of maintaining such a clinical dietetics management information system outweigh its cost and shortcomings.

Conclusion

The directors of clinical dietary services and food service administrators are facing increasing demands for dietary services from physicians as well as from patients and their families. To effectively evaluate this increased demand, it is imperative that current levels of care be defined and a methodology for evaluating requests for additional nutritional care be developed. These objectives may be met by establishing a standing committee of the medical board that meets periodically to evaluate nutritional care. Concurrently, the changing hospital fiscal environment has caused hospital administrators to carefully review personnel allocation and assign resources to departments that can demonstrate need through accountability and attainment of acceptable productivity standards.

It is in the best interests of the patient that the clinical dietetic staff and the institution have well-defined and predetermined objectives, together with well-established procedures for job accountability and valid measures for productivity. This process requires the food service administrator to maintain adequate records that support the proper management of the department. There is no substitute for applying sound management practice.

Notes

[1] Headlines. Less money ahead, McMahon warns. *Hospitals.* 55:18, July 16, 1981.

[2] Joint Commission on Accreditation of Hospitals. *Accreditation Manual for Hospitals.* Chicago: JCAH, 1982.

[3] Becker, D. S., and Kaud, F. A. A study of the clinical dietetics staff performance measurement technique. Unpublished study, May 1979.

[4] Walters, F. M., and others. Optimal nutritional care/cost equation—a proposal. *Journal of the American Dietetic Association.* 61:165, Aug. 1972.

[5] Kaud, F. A. Food Service Department financial statement. Paper presented at a workshop of the American Society for Hospital Food Service Administrators of the American Hospital Association, Denver, July 16-17, 1979.

[6] Becker, D. S., and Kaud, F. A. A study of the clinical dietetics staff performance measurement techniques. Madison, WI: University of Wisconsin Hospital and Clinics. Unpublished study, Feb. 1981.

[7] Becker, D. S. Productivity measurement methods for clinical dietetics. In: *1979 Abstracts,* Proceedings of the Annual Meeting of the American Dietetic Association, Chicago: ADA, 1979.

[8] Colorado and Denver Dietetic Associations. *Standards of Practice—Nutritional Quality Assurance in Acute Care Hospitals.* Denver, CO: Colorado and Denver Dietetic Associations, 1980.

[9] The American Dietetic Association. *A Report of the Professional Standards Review Committee.* Chicago: ADA, 1976.

[10] Schiller, R. S., and Behm, V. Auditing Dietetic Services. *Hospitals.* 53:122, Apr. 16, 1979.

Figure 10. Example of Objectives and Tasks for a Clinical Inpatient Dietitian

Percentage of Time	Employee goals and activities
48	**Provision of nutritional care to all patients on assigned units** ■ Obtains nutrition histories. Reviews pertinent medical data and makes assessments to determine nutritional status ■ Assesses appropriateness of diet orders ■ Develops appropriate nutrition care plan, monitors its implementation, and evaluates the effectiveness of the care plan ■ Makes rounds of all patients on a medical unit, as assigned during the two meal services daily, and evaluates patients' ability to consume food, reviews patients' knowledge of diet/nutrition, evaluates meal service, and so forth ■ Attends and actively participates in interdisciplinary rounds and conferences
15	**Provision of patient education** ■ Provides patients with instructional materials, and instructs patients on their diet utilizing available resources ■ Follows up with patients on diet information and menu selection ■ Prepares nutrition referrals and follows up through local calls and/or letters. Acts as a nutritional resource person for members of the health care team and the community
15	**Records in medical record** ■ Records pertinent information in the patient's medical record
10	**Menu review for nutritional adequacy** ■ Reviews menus for nutritional adequacy ■ Writes menus for modified diets when appropriate
12	**Other activities** ■ Participates in professional development activities ■ Participates in the education of dietetic interns, technicians, and so forth ■ Conducts educational programs for hospital staff and the community ■ Attends weekly staff meetings for dietitians and departmental meetings ■ Participates in quality assurance, and reviews policy and procedures as assigned ■ Prepares reports ■ Performs any other duties as assigned by supervisors

Source: Becker, D.S., and Kaud, F.A. A Study of the clinical dietetics staff performance measurement technique. Unpublished study, February 1981.

Figure 11. Example of Objectives and Tasks for a Dietetic Technician

Percentage of Time	Employee Goals and Activities
60	**Review of menus of assigned patients for nutritional adequacy** ■ Aids patients in menu selections, reviewing menus of all patients on nursing units assigned for nutritional adequacy assessment and adherence to dietary orders ■ Writes menus that adhere to patients dietary orders, food preference, and diet patterns and that provide nutritional adequacy
25	**Provision of nutritional care to patients assigned** ■ Makes rounds of patients at two meal services daily to ascertain quality of food and service and patients' ability to consume food, performs visual assessment of patients, and initiates communications and/or actions as determined by observation ■ Interviews patients as assigned to determine food preferences ■ Consults with the dietitian regarding nutritional care of patients, and reports progress of patients to the dietitian ■ Assists the dietitian in planning an individualized pattern for patients in accordance with dietary modifications. Responsible for this information being recorded in departmental records
5	**Provision of appropriate nutrition information in patient medical records** ■ Records nutritional information in patients' medical records as assigned by supervisor
5	**Utilization of teaching aids and educational techniques for individualized instructions of patient and family** ■ Instructs patients and their family on the diets ordered and general nutrition principles ■ Helps develop and assess teaching tools and instructional materials
5	**Participation in department meetings and educational programs** ■ Participates in staff meetings ■ Participates in in-service education programs ■ Prepares and presents, under supervision, educational programs to the staff and community ■ Performs any other duties as assigned by supervisor

Source: Becker, D.S., and Kaud, F.A. A study of the clinical dietetics staff performance measurement technique. Unpublished study, February 1981.

Figure 12. Example of Relative Value Unit Calculations for the Clinical Inpatient Dietitian

Activities	RVU
Nutrition assessment (patient visitation, reviewing medical records, and so forth)	
■ Basic (plastic surgery, appendectomy)	1.0
■ Intermediate (obesity, diabetes mellitus)	3.0
■ Complex (burn patient–over 20% TBS, renal failure, patient receiving TPN, major trauma)	3.0
Menus	
■ Review house diet menus (general, soft)	0.25
■ Writing basic modified diets (90 mEq sodium, weight reduction, including patterns)	1.0
■ Writing complex modified diets (renal, gluten-free, diabetic-sodium restriction, including patterns)	1.5
Charting in patients' medical records	
■ Basic (general)	1.0
■ Intermediate (weight reduction)	1.5
■ Complex (renal, TPN)	3.0
Counseling	
■ Basic (general nutrition questions, no added salt)	1.5
■ Intermediate (weight reduction, refresher for diabetic, 90 mEq sodium)	3.5
■ Complex (renal, newly diagnosed diabetic)	4.0
Interaction with other health care team members	
■ Intermediate (weight reduction, 90 mEq sodium)	1.0
■ Complex (renal, TPN, tube feeding)	3.0
Evaluation of meal service	0.25
Continuing education	0.01

Source: Becker, D.S., and Kaud, F.A. A study of clinical dietetics staff performance measurement technique. Unpublished study, May 1979.

Note: 1.0 RVU = 10 minutes.

Figure 13. Sample Form for Clinical Dietetics Weekly Status Report

Date _____
Report of _____

Clinical Dietetics
Weekly Status Report

Number of Patients Visited

Units	Monday	Tuesday	Wednesday	Thursday	Friday

Diets Written

Units	Mon.	Tues.	Wed.	Thur.	Fri.	Total
Total						

Diets Checked

Units	Mon.	Tues.	Wed.	Thur.	Fri.	Total
Total						

Education

Date	Topic	Speaker	Time	Date	Topic	Speaker	Time

Teaching

Date	Topic	Group	No. Attended	Time	Date	Topic	Group	No. Attended	Time

Meetings

Date	Group	Purpose	Time	Date	Group	Purpose	Time

Interdisciplinary Rounds

Date	Group	No. of Points Discussed	Time	Date	Group	No. of Points Discussed	Time

Record Keeping

Date	Activity	Time	Date	Activity	Time

Projects

Date	Activity	Time	Date	Activity	Time

Nonroutine Activities

Date	Activity	Time	Date	Activity	Time

Figure 13 (continued)

Clinical Dietetics Weekly Status Report

Date _____
Report of _____

Date	Unit/Room No.	Patient's Name	Diet Type	Consulted with Staff	Read Chart	Prep.	Counseling	Charting	Referral

Developed by D.S. Becker, F.A. Kaud, and S. Crocket.

Figure 14. Sample Form for Diet Status Report

Diet Status Report

Unit _____   Date _____

Room No.	Name	Diet	Dinner	Breakfast	Lunch	Remarks

Note: This form is prepared in quadruplicate; one copy to accompany each meal and one copy for the nursing file.

Figure 15. Sample Report of a Clinical Dietetics Staff's Weekly Activities, Based on Time-Task Allocation Analysis

Major Responsibilities	Hours Worked per Week	Total	Percentage of Time
Nutrition assessment			
■ Patient visitation	97.6		
■ Medical record review	46.8		
■ Interdisciplinary patient care conferences and consultations with staff	27.0		
■ Preparation time	14.0		
		185.4	32
Menu review for nutritional adequacy			
■ Menu written	120.6		
■ Menu reviewed	53.5		
		174.1	30
Charting in the medical record		63.5	11
Patient Education			
■ Patient instruction and follow-up	57.2		
■ Referral	1.0		
		58.2	10
Job related activities (education, teaching, meetings, record keeping, projects, and so forth		95.0	16
		576.2	99

Source: Becker, D.S., and Kaud, F.A. A study of clinical dietetics staff performance measurement techniques. Unpublished study, Feb. 1981.

Figure 16. Sample Report of a Dietitian's Weekly Activities in an Outpatient Nutrition Clinic, Based on Time-Task Allocation Analysis

Major Responsibilities	Hours Worked per Week[a]	Percentage of Time
Counseling (one-to-one and group)	24.0	60
Charting in the medical record	6.0	15
Participating with the health care team	4.0	10
Community programs	4.0	10
Other activities: publication of newsletter, training programs, and so forth	1.2	3
Continuing education	0.8	2
	40.0	100

Source: Becker, D.S., and Kaud, F.A. A study of clinical dietetics staff performance measurement techniques. Unpublished study, May 1979.

[a]Two 15-minute breaks per day were included in the calculation.

Figure 17. Example of a Weekly Activities Budget Study for an Inpatient Clinical Dietetics Department

A. Actual Activities

Major Responsibilities	1980-81: Actual					1981-82: Actual				
	Number of Activities	Hours Worked	Percentage of Patient Days	Percentage of Admissions	Number of Activities	Hours Worked	Percentage of Patient Days	Percentage of Admissions
A. Nutritional assessment								
1. Patient visitation	2,537	84.6	88		2,929	97.6	98	
2. Patient's medical records reviewed	136	22.6		33	162.6	27.1		38
3. Patient care conferences		15.0				23.0		
4. Preparation time		13.9				13.6		
B. Patient education								
1. Patient instruction	242	54.7			280	57.4		
2. Written referral	8	1.5		2.3	6	0.7		1.8
C. Charting in patient medical records	115	22.8		28	170	33.2		40
D. Menus evaluated for nutritional adequacy								
1. Menus written	1,020	119	35		890	103.8	31	
2. Menus reviewed	1,270	42.3	44		1,327	44.2	46	
Subtotal	2,290	161.3	79		2,217	148.0	77	
E. Other activities (in-service education, interns' class time, meetings, projects, and so on)		113.9				116.1		
F. Total hours worked		490.3				516.7		
G. Hours paid		486.8				557.6		
H. Number of FTEs	12.28				13.94			

Management of the Clinical Dietetics Staff ■ 75

Figure 17. (continued)

B. Estimated Activities

Major Responsibilities	1982-83: Estimate Current Staffing				1982-83: Estimate Improved Service			
	Number of Activities	Hours Worked	Percentage of Patient Days	Percentage of Admissions	Number of Activities	Hours Worked	Percentage of Patient Days	Percentage of Admissions
A. Nutritional assessment								
1. Patient visitation	2,900	97.6	98		2,900	97.6	98	
2. Patient's medical records reviewed	300	35.0		70	401	46.8		95
3. Patient Care conferences		23.0				27.0		
4. Preparation time		14.0				14.0		
B. Patient education								
1. Patient instruction	286	57.2			286	57.2		
2. Written referral	8	1.0		2.3	8	1.0		2.3
C. Charting in patient medical records	290	48.8		68	401	63.5		95
D. Menus evaluated for nutritional adequacy								
1. Menus written	1,034	120.6	35		1,034	120.6	35	
2. Menus reviewed	1,200	40.0	41		1,605	53.5	54	
Subtotal	2,234	160.6	76		2,639	174.1	89	
E. Other activities (in-service education, interns' class time, meetings, projects, and so forth)		95.0				95.0		
F. Total hours worked		532.2				576.2		
G. Hours paid								
H. Number of FTEs	14.92				15.8			

Figure 17. (continued)

C. Productivity Measures of Selected Activities

Major Responsibilities	Actual 1980-81 (Minutes/Task)	Actual 1981-82 (Minutes/Task)	Estimate Current Staff for 1982-83 (Minutes/Task)	Estimate Improved Service for 1982-83 (Minutes/Task)
A. Patients' medical records reviewed	10	10	7	7
B. Patient education[a]	13.5	12.5	12	12
C. Charting in patient medical records	11.9	11.7	10.1	9.5

Prepared by D.S. Becker. Data include work performed by clinical dietitians, dietetic technicians, and dietetic interns during clinical rotation.

[a]The education philosophy of this hospital is that numerous short instructions per patient are more effective than one long instruction.

Management of the Clinical Dietetics Staff ■ 77